TESTOSTERONE
IS
YOUR FRIEND

A Book for Men and Women

Roger Mason

Testosterone Is Your Friend
by
Roger Mason

ISBN   1884820-74-3
Library of Congress Catalog Number: 2001012345
Categories: 1. Health 2. Nutrition
Printed in the U.S.A.
1st Printing Fall 2004

Published by Safe Goods
561 Shunpike Rd.
Sheffield, MA 01257
(413) 229-7935
www.safegoodspub.com

Contents

About This Book

This is the only real book in the world that factually and accurately talks about testosterone for men and women. You will find countless journal citations so you will know that everything you are reading is heavily documented by published international research. It is only in the last few years that we have finally learned very much about testosterone — especially for women. Until recently nearly all research was done with toxic oral and injected salts instead of real, natural testosterone used sublingually and transdermally. The worldwide medical profession walks in darkness here. Most people depend on doctors for their ailments, but doctors just cannot help you when it comes to hormones — and that includes naturopaths, gynecologists, life extension specialists and even endocrinologists.

Testosterone is not a Magic Hormone to be used by itself to cure what ails you. All our hormones work together in concert, and all of them must be balanced together in endocrine harmony. This means you need to test and balance your basic fourteen hormones as much as possible to get the best results. The last chapter "Your Other Hormones" is the most important one to read.

Hormones are only one part of a total natural lifestyle. Diet is everything and hormonal balance is secondary. You should eat a whole grain based, low fat, high fiber diet. Supplements are important, and anyone over the age of forty should be taking at least a dozen natural supplements. Regular exercise is a pillar of staying healthy all your life. Avoiding (at least limiting) bad habits is a big part of this. Fasting is the most powerful healing method known. Lastly, meditation and prayer keep your spiritual house in order. Men should read my book "The Natural Prostate Cure" and women should read my "No More Horse Estrogen!" Everyone should read my "Zen Macrobiotics for Americans" to learn more about diet, supplements, and hormones in general. The best doctor you can have is yourself.

Overview

Our hormones are most basic to our health and well being, yet almost no one knows anything about their own hormone levels. Medical doctors know almost nothing about our hormones, and that includes endocrinologists who are supposed to specialize in such. Doctors rarely test for hormone levels and even then only for one or two. Doctors generally don't know how to properly test hormone levels, which hormones to test for, or what the ranges should be, much less how to administer them or in what forms.

You can direct your doctor as to precisely which free, unbound hormones you want tested and see your own results. You can also test most hormones yourself with saliva and not use a doctor. Testosterone is one of the most important human hormones for both men and women, yet proper testosterone supplementation is almost unknown to the medical profession, especially for women. Low testosterone levels cause countless problems for both sexes including decreased libido, sexual dysfunction, less sexual satisfaction, infertility, irritability, depression, poor concentration, decreased sense of well being, prostate disease and testicular decline in men, diabetes and other blood sugar problems, gynecological conditions in women, impaired cognition, less stamina, obesity, high body mass index, decreased muscle mass, gynecomastia and smaller penis size in men, impaired vasomotor function, osteoporosis, coronary heart problems, diseases of all kinds, and conditions we still haven't researched. All in all we're talking about not merely longer lifespan, but a better all around *quality* of life by maintaining youthful levels.

It is only in the last few years that scientists have started to use natural sublingual and transdermal testosterone rather than unnatural toxic oral and injected salts. The pharmaceutical corporations are still trying to push injectable ester salts, overpriced patches, and implanted pellets instead of inexpensive creams, gels, and sublingual solutions. In fact, the currently available gels are very weak and vastly overpriced. One dollar's worth of testosterone will often retail for one hundred dollars in a cream or gel. Sublingual solutions are unheard of. Severely overcharging for natural hormones is nothing short of criminal.

Men can suffer from deficient testosterone at any age, but usually only after the age of forty or so. Men cannot naturally overproduce testosterone or suffer from hypergonadism. Real life testing shows that literally 90 percent of men over age fifty can and should use supplemental testosterone to maintain youthful levels.

Women can suffer from deficient or excessive testosterone at any age even in their teenage years. Most women don't even know they have testosterone in the bodies much less know their level! Doctors generally have no idea women need to maintain youthful levels of this, and consider testosterone "the male hormone". We need much more research on women here.

There are many hundreds of studies in my files and this book could be a lot, lot longer. Half of this book would be devoted to and should be devoted to women, but the research just isn't there. At least 95 percent of all testosterone research is done on men only. In the future we'll have far more research on the androgens testosterone, DHEA and androstenedione for women. Meanwhile the women reading this book should just generally realize the benefits discussed basically apply to them as well.

Chapter 1: What Is Testosterone?

Men and women have exactly the same hormones only in different amounts. There are three basic androgens, which include testosterone, androstenedione and DHEA. Men produce about 6-8 milligrams per day of testosterone while women produce about one twentieth of that (approximately 300 micrograms). Women do have about one tenth the blood level men have as they retain it more efficiently. Men produce testosterone in their testicles and adrenal glands and cannot naturally overproduce this hormone. There is no such condition as "hypergonadism" in men. The only way men can have an excessive level is by taking some type of testosterone supplement. Even then the male body will only allow so much blood testosterone, and then turns any excess into estradiol and estrone. This is done by "aromatization" using the enzyme 5-alpha reductase. Androstenedione levels (and androstenediol) generally parallel that of testosterone. DHEA can generally be too low, and only rarely too high in men as they age.

Women produce testosterone basically with their ovaries and adrenal glands. Prior to menopause they can and do sometimes overproduce this and suffer from "androgenicity". After menopause levels generally fall, but hypertestosterone levels are still possible even after a hysterectomy. Excessive testosterone levels can cause serious problems in women such as polycystic ovaries (PCOS) and hirstutism (excessive hair growth). Androstenedione levels should also be monitored in women since they can also be too high. Excessive DHEA levels in women can contribute to androgenicity as well. One third of American women are unnecessarily butchered by the medical profession and have their uterus cut out. The ovaries *always* atrophy and die after a hysterectomy despite the constant denials by the doctors. Let's repeat that - the ovaries *always* die after hysterectomy. This means one third of women over the age of forty have their hormone levels seriously disrupted and their entire endocrine (hormone) system completely out of line. Ladies, please read my book *No More Horse Estrogen!*

9

Most all of the research on testosterone is done on males since this is erroneously considered "the male hormone". Just because men have ten times blood hormone does not make it any less important in women. Until more research is done on women we must logically concur that the male studies basically apply to women as well. The medical profession knows little about testosterone or any other hormone. This includes urologists, gynecologists, naturopaths, life extension specialists, and even endocrinologists! This kind of ignorance is simply inexcusable.

Recently published international clinical literature overwhelmingly proves how vital youthful testosterone levels are to both men and women for countless reasons. Doctors almost never test testosterone (or any other hormone) levels and have almost no idea how to test them or what to look for. Further, they have no idea how to raise testosterone levels safely, effectively and naturally. You must realize you *cannot* look to any medical professional for help in this area.

You are better off testing your own hormone levels with saliva testing kits, judging your results, and ordering any needed prescription hormones (such as testosterone, estriol, T3, and T4) from the Internet. It will be repeated over and over that all *your hormones work together* as a team and all your basic hormones must be in balance for any of them to be as effective as possible. Please read chapter 17 "Your Other Hormones" carefully.

$C_{19}H_{28}O_2$

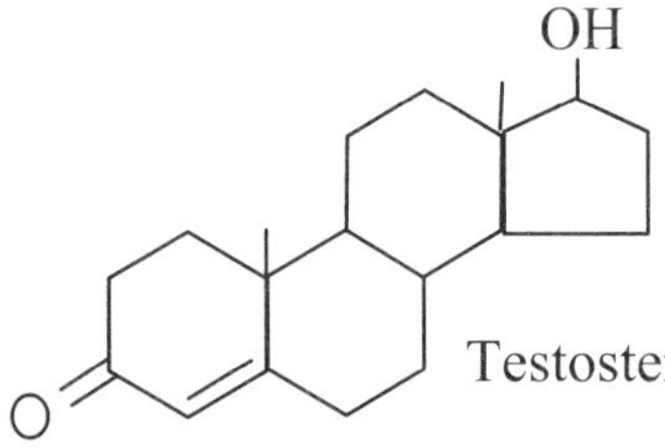

Testosterone, CAS 58-22-0

17 beta-hydroxy-4-androsten-3-one   mol. wt. 288.41

Chapter 2: Androstenedione and Precursors

There are a variety of supposed testosterone precursors available including muira puama, homeopathic testosterone, Lepidium root, Tribulus terrestis, zinc formulations, tongkat ali (Longifolium), various herbal combinations, and other such concoctions that have shown to be useless for this purpose. Studies prove that *none* of these have any value whatsoever and are simply well advertised scams. The only precursors that have any possible potential value are the androstenedione family.

Androstendedione and androstenediol are the direct precursors of testosterone in mammals. These exist naturally in the 4-position structurally. There are also many analogs of these including 5- position, 19- position and nor- analogs. The only ones that have any science at all behind them are plain old, regular 4-positioned androstenedione or androstenediol. There has been an endless parade of junk science studies that purport to show how "dangerous" androstenedione is and how "ineffective" it is in raising testosterone in humans. In nearly every single one of these "studies" young men with naturally high testosterone are given huge overdoses of hundreds of milligrams of androstenedione. Even the few "studies" that used middle-aged men were not hypogonadal and were still heavily overdosed. Since men cannot normally have high levels this overdose simply raises estrogen and estrone. Testosterone is not raised — just estrogens! Amazingly there have been no published studies on the responsible low-dose (i.e. 50 mg or less) use of androstenedione in hypogonadal men anywhere in the world, much less on testosterone deficient women. Women have ovaries rather than testicles and metabolize androstenedione (and androstenediol) into testosterone more efficiently than men. It may well be possible for women to take oral androstenedione to raise their testosterone, but we will need studies to see if their blood levels of androstenedione go up too much and if any excess estrone and estradiol are formed as by-products. Since one third of American women are castrated (hysterectomy) without cause and their testosterone levels are cut in half, this would certainly be much needed research.

The University of Ontario was about the only institution in the world to even address this issue (Canadian Journal of Applied Physiology v. 27, 2002, pp. 628-45). They pointed out that sublingual administration of the androstenedione family is far more effective in hypogonadal men. It is very difficult to solubilize androstenedione and it must be complexed in cyclodextrin suspension to dissolve under the tongue. They referred to Blacquier et al back in 1967 (Acta Endocrinologica v. 55, pp.697-704) who found that androstenediol was almost three times as effective in transforming into testosterone than androstenedione. If this is true we should be studying androstenediol rather than androstenedione primarily in both men and women. They also referred to Horton et al back in 1955 (Journal of Clinical Investigation v. 45, pp. 301-13) who was one of the only researchers in the world to show that women transform the androstenedione family into testosterone more efficiently than men. They found that about 60 percent of plasma testosterone is derived from androstenedione biologically in women, while only about 37 percent is derived in men.

They referred to Mahesh et al, back in 1962 (Acta Endocrinologica v. 41, pp. 400-6) where women were given completely irresponsible 100 mg doses of oral androstenedione and then 100 mg of DHEA! They also found orally administered androstenedione family hormones were very poorly absorbed by either sex, and intravenously administration was far more effective. Of course, injecting people with anything is always a poor idea unless absolutely necessary in a medical emergency. We must always remember that women only make about 300 mcg (less than one third of one milligram) of testosterone daily and a general rule is to get about 150 mcg into their blood if they are proven to be deficient. While this is the best review ever published on testosterone prohormones, they still just didn't comprehend that high dose oral supplementation, especially in young men, is completely irrational and merely produces estrogens. They continually referred to previous studies where healthy men with normally high testosterone levels were given irrational amounts of oral androstenedione. Again, men only produce about 6-8 mg a day of testosterone and men with normal levels should not take any at all. King et al in 1999 gave healthy young men 300 mg of oral androstenedione. Of course their estradiol and estrone levels rose dramatically, but not their testosterone. Wallace et al gave middle-aged men both 100 mg of DHEA and 100 mg of androstenedione, but did not even test them to see if they were deficient in either hormone!

Leder et al in 2000 gave healthy men 300 mg of androstenedione and got huge rises in both estradiol and estrone, but not testosterone. Earnest et al in 2000 gave men either 200 mg of androstenedione or androstenediol who were not low in testosterone. At least Earnest found out that the androstenediol was more effective than the androstenedione. Ballantyne et al gave healthy men 200 mg of oral androstenedione with the usual bad effects. Brown et al in 2000 gave men 300 mg of oral androstenedione and got estrogens. The list goes on. There has not been one single study giving hypogonadal middle aged or elderly men a reasonable 50 mg oral dose of any of the androstenedione prohormones, much less using the more promising androstenediol, much less using this sublingually in suspension. These completely unscientific "studies" will now be used to ban all the androstenedione family and make mere possession a felony punishable by five years in federal prison under the Steroid Hormone Act.

When androstenedione first became available in the marketplace in the mid-1990's many older men successfully used this to raise testosterone levels by simply taking an inexpensive 50 mg tablet. At the time this seemed like a practical and effective means of raising testosterone without seeing a doctor to get a prescription. It should be mentioned that unreputable companies tried to promote supposedly transdermal androstenedione creams, which were claimed to penetrate the skin and bypass the liver to make it more effective. These were plain and simple frauds, yet you still see them offered from time to time. Androstenedione and androstenediol are not metabolized into testosterone very effectively whether taken orally, or used transdermally. Injections are more effective but very ill advised. If you used, for example, a ridiculous 5 grams of 10 percent androstenedione cream (which would be 500 mg of actual androstenedione), you would only be getting about 50 mg of actual hormone into your bloodstream (a 10% absorption rate is reasonably expected here). With an 8 percent conversion rate you would be getting a mere 4 mg of actual testosterone in your body. That means at best that 500 mg of androstenedione would end up as a mere 4 mg of available testosterone in your blood - ideally and theoretically that is. We simply don't know what would happen with women. Since women only produce about 300 mcg (one third of one mg) of testosterone a day it would be reasonable to experiment with using a half gram of 10 percent androstenedione cream on women who are low in testosterone. This might not work at all, however. Again, the research on women is ignored.

One possible answer here that has received almost no attention is to use the sublingual route especially with androstenediol rather than androstenedione. It is very difficult to dissolve any of the androstenedione family unfortunately. This can be done by cyclodextrin suspension, but only in a laboratory and not at home. Research into low dose sublingual administration of androstenediol for both men and women might turn out to be very beneficial.

One problem is that some men simply don't metabolize oral supplemental androstenedione into testosterone and they just make estrogens from it. The biggest problem is, that after a period of time, the androstenedione is no longer effective and will not make testosterone. No matter how you choose to raise your testosterone you must monitor your estrone and estradiol before you start. Then you should monitor your levels every 6 months to make sure you aren't raising your estrogens. Even if androstenedione does work for a man, and even if he is willing to monitor his estradiol and estrone every six months, it will simply stop working after a while. Obviously this just isn't the long-term answer.

Another concern is that young body builders with diminished intelligence were reading articles and advertisements in the

14

body building magazines. They would then take very large doses of androstenedione up to several hundred milligrams per day. Since they already had high, youthful levels of testosterone they were simply raising their estradiol and estrone levels dangerously and not making any testosterone at all. Worse, they were putting themselves at risk for various forms of cancer and other serious conditions. This made the politicians jump on the legislative bandwagon to ban over the counter sales of androstenedione without a prescription. House Bill 207, Senate Bill 502, etc. are not anti-andro bills at all, but rather *antisupplement* bills that will open the door to take away your rights to buy all natural hormones and supplements. There is no doubt androstenedione (as happened with the natural plant stimulant ephedrine) will soon be felony classified as an illegal drug. Then, all the natural hormones such as DHEA, melatonin, pregnenolone and progesterone will also be classified as dangerous drugs with long prison sentences for mere possession as is true in Canada and other countries.

One answer to this for both men and women is to find a medical doctor who is well educated in testosterone therapy. You can talk to your local compounding pharmacist and ask him which doctors are writing prescriptions for transdermal testosterone. Then ask him if he will make up a sublingual testosterone solution for you. The problem here is the doctor will want an office visit, an expensive blood test, a second office visit, and an expensive compounded testosterone product from the compounding pharmacist. Often the doctor won't even make the prescription refillable. Later he'll want more office visits and blood tests to continue your therapy. This is obviously the road to the poor house.

There are Internet sites selling both sublingual testosterone tablets and aqueous suspensions of natural testosterone. In the U.S. it is perfectly legal for you under U.S. Code 21, Section 331 to order (use registered mail) or personally import drugs from foreign countries for your own use. The problem is when you go to these Internet sites you'll probably be confused by the array of scams such as homeopathic transdermal testosterone cream and the endless variety of dangerous weightlifter steroids offered.

15

The bottom line here is that androstenedione and andro-stenediol cannot be recommended long term for men for the following reasons: the conversion is poor; the effects are temporary; some men don't convert to testosterone at all; the risks of estrogen formation are high; it will soon be illegal; and constant blood or saliva monitoring is necessary. For women we simply do not know what happens when they take oral androstenedione family pro-hormones, use transdermal cream, or use them sublingually. This would be most interesting to investigate. One study at King's College in London (Clinical Chemistry v. 49, 2003, pp. 167-9) gave women a toxic 100 mg of oral androstenedione, which drove their testosterone levels through the roof! Five milligrams would have been a reasonable investigative dose, but only in women proven to be deficient in testosterone, which these women were not at all.

If you merely add a hydrogen atom to androstenedione you get testosterone. If you merely remove a hydrogen atom from an-drostenediol you also get testosterone. Both of these are the direct biological precursors in mammals.

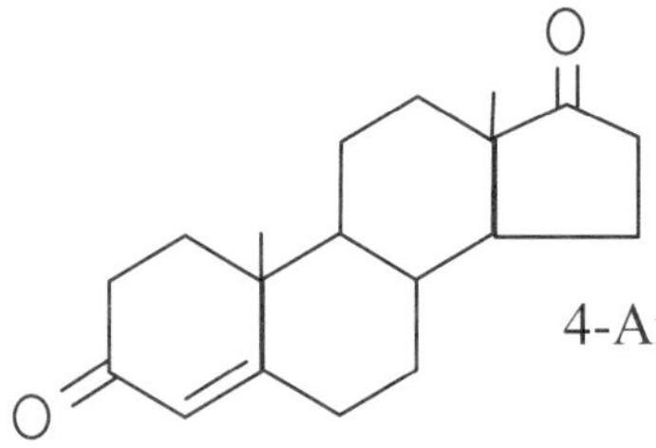

4-Androstenedione

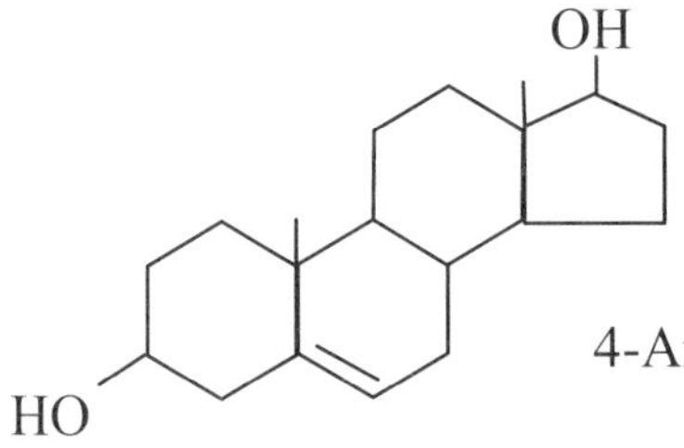

4-Androstenediol

Chapter 3: What Is Your Level?

Ideally you would want to know the levels of your fourteen (14) basic hormones. You will never enjoy the best of health until all your basic hormones are at youthful levels. There are two ways to test your free biological testosterone level. One, you can get your blood tested by a physician. This is expensive, requires office visits, and is completely unnecessary. Medical doctors basically know little about testosterone (or any other hormone), what it does, how to measure it, what the lab results mean, or the best delivery methods for men much less women. Two, you can simply test your own level by using a saliva testing lab. These saliva kits are readily available on the Internet and should be in the chain drug stores and pharmacies soon. You can pay as little as $25 per hormone to test your testosterone, pregnenolone, DHEA, melatonin, estradiol, estrone, estriol, progesterone, T3, T4, insulin, cortisol, or androstenedione. In 2004 you still have to use blood analysis for growth hormone. You can (man or woman) also check such other hormones as prolactin, LH and FSH. You simply send in a saliva sample to be analyzed by RIA (radioimmunoassay). You don't need a doctor, but California, New York, and Ohio ban people from doing this! The medical profession does not want you to have any freedom whatsoever for self-diagnosis or self-medication. The fact that three states (so far) have outlawed testing your own saliva should horrify you. More states will soon follow due to pressure from the medical profession. If you live in these states simply have your results sent to a friend or relative in another state to get around such unconstitutional, irrational, and ridiculous laws.

Measuring free, bioavailable, unbound hormones using saliva has been known to scientists for over two decades now. In the last few years it has finally been brought to the consumer. This is one of the greatest technological breakthroughs in medicine, but is still relatively unknown. Doctors at Georgia State University proved the validity and reliability of saliva hormone testing in 1995 (Clinical Chemistry v. 41, pp. 1581-4). They compared results from nine laboratories in four countries using 100 men and 100 women. Basically the results were very consistent and reliable. There were some unacceptable variations from a few of the labs, which means you have to use a reliable, well established testing facility with a good reputation.

You will hear some popular and well known, but un-enlightened advocates recommending urine testing to determine your hormone levels. Urine is a waste product and tells us what the body doesn't want and is excreting. The only possible rare use for urine diagnosis is to compare the excretion of various hormones with the blood or saliva levels. (The same holds true with toxic elements like mercury or cadmium, which require actual blood diagnosis). A 1995 study from the Chinese University in Hong Kong (Clinica Chimica Acta. v. 236, pp. 87-92) proves this. Healthy, normal men were tested for their testosterone and estradiol levels both by blood and urine. They did not find a good correlation at all between these, and stated, "Serum estradiol showed no significant correlation." As men age their blood and saliva estradriol and estrone (but not their estriol) levels go up dramatically, but not their excretion of these estrogens. If anyone recommends urine testing for your hormones you know they have no idea what they are talking about.

When doctors measure your serum or plasma blood levels they usually test your total testosterone, your bound testosterone, sometimes your free testosterone and then calculate a total-to-free ratio, as if that has some important, esoteric meaning. Not only is this inexcusable ignorance on their part, but it is also a fine way to make money by giving patients tests they don't need and that do not help them. If you have your sex hormones tested you only want your *free*, unbound, biologically available level tested. About 98 to 99 percent of testosterone is bound to SHBG (sex hormone binding globulin) and albumin and is biologically unavailable. Testing your bound and total testosterone levels tells you almost nothing and is a waste of time and money. Just test your *free*, unbound levels of sex hormones.

Surprisingly you usually cannot compare levels from one lab to another except by general terms such as "low normal" or "below range". Whether you test your blood or saliva you cannot take those numbers and compare them to another lab unless they have the exact same range. There is simply no way to convert saliva results to blood results or vice versa. Just go by whether your results are low or high according to the given range.

Testosterone is a very powerful hormone and you absolutely cannot use it unless you first prove you have low normal levels or below normal levels. Medical doctors generally tell you that you're fine if your hormone levels are "in range" for your age. This is not true at all. The ideal is *youthful* level you had at about age thirty. Youthful levels are the key to good health and life extension. If you are seventy you certainly don't want the same levels as all the other seventy-year olds, do you? It is important to realize that men and women who are vegetarians, or who eat seafood, and do not eat red meat and dairy foods, have lower levels of sex hormones than carnivores. You can see by the charts that both men and women generally have lower testosterone levels as they age.

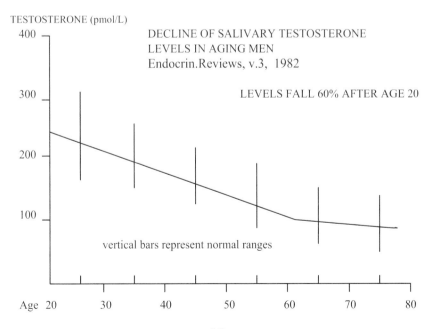

TESTOSTERONE (pmol/L)

DECLINE OF SALIVARY TESTOSTERONE LEVELS IN AGING MEN
Endocrin.Reviews, v.3, 1982

LEVELS FALL 60% AFTER AGE 20

vertical bars represent normal ranges

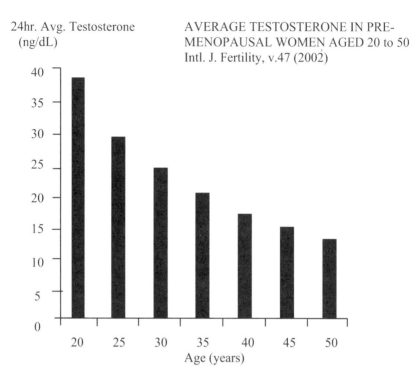

24hr. Avg. Testosterone (ng/dL)

AVERAGE TESTOSTERONE IN PRE-MENOPAUSAL WOMEN AGED 20 to 50
Intl. J. Fertility, v.47 (2002)

Age (years)

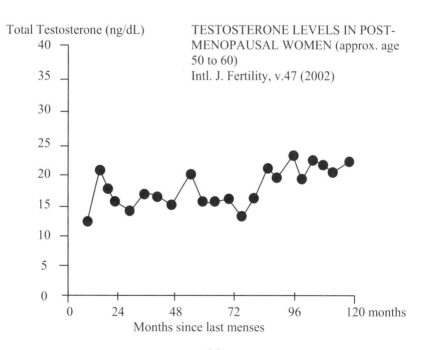

Total Testosterone (ng/dL)

TESTOSTERONE LEVELS IN POST-MENOPAUSAL WOMEN (approx. age 50 to 60)
Intl. J. Fertility, v.47 (2002)

Months since last menses

Chapter 4: How Do I Use It?

Basically the only safe, inexpensive and effective way to use natural testosterone is either by a sublingual (under the tongue) solution or a transdermal cream or gel. (DMSO transdermal solutions are not approved by the FDA- DMSO is a solvent that transfers drugs through the skin.) "Natural" means free testosterone that is not in a synthetic salted ester form such as propionate, enanthate or undecanoate. Most ignorant, "uneducated" physicians still use toxic methyl testosterone. In fact, the most common testosterone prescribed for American women is methyl testosterone! This is proof the medical profession walks in darkness. The very few medical doctors who do administer testosterone generally use oral (not sublingual) or i.m. (intramuscular) injected toxic ester salts. You do not want to take these dangerous and unnatural forms by mouth or by hypodermic needle. In the next chapter you'll see that patches are very overpriced and have poor permeation.

Surgically implanted pellets may be natural testosterone, but are expensive, very impractical and totally unnecessary. Oral testosterone salts are barely absorbed at all by the digestive system and produce over 97 percent unwanted and harmful metabolites. A testosterone nasal spray is not allowed by the FDA and cannot be purchased or even legally custom made by a compounding pharmacist (you could make your own, but this would be very difficult for the layman). Sublingual testosterone can be formulated in a vegetable oil solution by a compounding pharmacist to yield about 3-5 mg per drop to men and about 0.15 - 0.30 mg (150 to 300 mcg) per drop to women. Twenty-milligram sublingual tablets are available on the Internet as well and can be quartered to make them five milligram (these are too strong for women) and then used only five days a week (i.e. 25 mg per week). Adding DMSO (dimethylsulfoxide) to testosterone is also not approved by the FDA and cannot legally be sold or custom compounded. DMSO is a naturally occuring solvent that transfers any drug dissolved in it through your skin with over a 95 percent effectiveness.

You can, however, make up your own DMSO solution very easily. If you can get a water suspension of testosterone and evaporate it to powder, you would simply add 200 drops of DMSO to every gram (1,000 mg). This would give men 5 mg per day with about a 95 percent penetration. Adding 250 drops would give 4 mg per day, and adding 333 drops would give 3 mg a day. Women could use 100 mg of testosterone powder with 500 drops of DMSO to yield 0.2 mg (200 mcg) per day for almost a year and a half. Always keep these solutions refrigerated or frozen.

Please realize you are only going to raise your testosterone with real prescription testosterone, or possibly temporarily with a true biological precursor such as androstenedione or androstenediol. Every year you will find new scams offered, especially on the Internet and in body building magazines. These promise to raise your testosterone with non-prescription supplements. Tribulus terrestis (puncture vine), Muira puama, zinc compounds, Tongkat ali, Lepidium root, various herbal mixtures and other such garbage are being sold to gullible, uneducated people.

As of 2003 weak, overpriced one-percent natural testosterone gels have appeared in the chain pharmacies. You do not want to use them as they are 1) too weak (e.g. 1.0%) for men, 2) too strong for women, and 3) too expensive for anyone. You must find a compounding pharmacist in your state and can get your cream or gel by mail if there are none near where you live. You can find compounding pharmacists on the Internet, in the phone book or by contacting the International Association of Compounding Pharmacists on the Internet at www.iacprx.org.

Men can get a prescription for 100 grams of a 3 percent cream or gel for under $100. Shop around until you get this price. Women can get a prescription for 100 grams of a 0.3 percent cream or gel and should pay less than $50 even though this is only one tenth of what a man would need and should cost about $10 in an ideal world.

It may not be approved by the FDA, but you can add an equal amount of 99 percent DMSO to your cream or gel for much better absorption. If you add 100 grams of DMSO to 100 grams of testo-sterone cream or gel you would still use the same half gram or less (even though it has been diluted 50%) as it is now half the strength, but twice as effective. This will now last twice as long at the same price. Always monitor your levels for safety.

Foreign pharmacies, especially the Mexican ones, legally offer hormones over the Internet. Under federal law U.S. Code 21, Section 331 you can import prescription drugs for your own personal use without a prescription. Sublingual 20 mg tablets (not to be confused with oral testosterone salts such as undecanoate) and water suspensions are sold there. If you buy an aqueous suspension of natural testosterone (not a salt) you can simply evaporate this and dissolve it in oil for sublingual use. If you evaporate 500 mg (10 ml X 50 mg per ml) just add 100 drops of vegetable oil to get 5 mg per drop (or 125 drops to get 4 mg, or 166 drops to get 3 mg). Women can add 1,600 drops of vegetable oil to get 0.3 mg (300 mcg) per drop and have a four-year supply. Keep this refrigerated. You can also use the same amount of 99 percent DMSO to dissolve the testosterone and you can use one drop per day on thin skin such as the inner wrist. Again, no doctor or pharmacist can legally prescribe DMSO solutions for transdermal use, but you can make your own.

How much transdermal creams or gels should you use? If a man (3%) or woman (0.3%) uses a quarter gram a day, their 100 gram tube will last over a year. A quarter gram is a good benchmark to start with. If you need more you can always use a half gram. Since you probably don't have a chemist's scale in your house how do you know what a quarter gram is? A quarter teaspoon of most creams or gels (or plain water or oil) weighs about one gram. Therefore you want to use one fourth of a quarter teaspoon - which comes out to *one sixteenth* of a teaspoon. Be clear that we are talking about one sixteenth of a teaspoon or sixteen daily doses per teaspoon. Take a level quarter teaspoon of cream or gel and divide it into four portions to see what a quarter gram dab

23

looks like. This is what you'll be starting out with as a benchmark to see if this is what you need. A half gram would therefore be *one eighth* of a teaspoon.

It will be repeated over and over in this book that while natural hormones are a vital cornerstone of our health, that they are very powerful and cannot be used casually. Before using any hormone you must test your levels to see if you are deficient and need supplementation. If you have an excessive level only diet and lifestyle will normalize this. Do not take toxic prescription drugs to lower your hormones, as the side effects will outweigh the benefits. If you find you are low in a hormone and take a supplement you cannot assume or guess a correct dose. Only monitoring your free blood or saliva level will tell you if the dose you are taking is the correct one for your individual and unique biological makeup. Further, after taking any hormone and finding the correct dose you must monitor this at least once a year since your body will be changing as you age. You cannot assume that the dose you are taking will have the same exact effect year after year as obviously it won't.

If you are over the age of fifty you might just assume you are low in testosterone, DHEA, pregnenolone, melatonin, growth hormone and other such hormones. This is not necessarily true. The scientific way to use natural hormones is to test your natural level to see if you need supplementation, take a rational dose for 30 to 60 days and then test your level again, and monitor your level at least once a year. If you cause excessive levels you will have a mirror image metabolic imbalance no different than with having deficient levels. Always remember you are looking for the *youthful* level you enjoyed at about the age of 30 years old. Hyper levels are pathological levels and cause serious harm much of which we have no clear understanding of yet.

Chapter 5: Various Delivery Systems

This is going to be a long and well-cited chapter for very good reasons. It must be shown conclusively that generally medical doctors — even in the most respected clinics, hospitals and universities - know almost nothing about supplemental testosterone (or any other hormones). Nearly all of the very few doctors who actually administer testosterone are doing it "bass ackwards" and aren't well educated as to what they're doing. Yes, this also includes the pricey life extension clinics. We're going to see what they are doing wrong. We're going to see why we shouldn't take unnatural esters either orally or by injections. We're going to see that low doses of plain natural testosterone administered transdermally or sublingually are the most practical, safest, most effective and least expensive ways to use it. (DMSO delivery is not allowed by law and hasn't been studied in clinics). Let's look at some studies on the various delivery systems to see what works, what doesn't work, and why.

You will also see why patches technically do work, but are a very overpriced promotion of the pharmaceutical corporations. Subcutaneously implanted time release pellets are natural testosterone, but are very expensive and have to be implanted surgically under the skin by a doctor. This is simply impractical and unnecessary. Even the new prescription hydroalcoholic gels sold in the chain pharmacies are weak and very overpriced. Most of the compounding pharmacists will try to vastly overcharge you for a transdermal cream that contains a mere two dollars worth (about 25 cents worth in the case of women) of actual natural testosterone. Finding a doctor who will even write a prescription for transdermal or sublingual testosterone from a compounding pharmacist can be very difficult. In 2004 we can hope that the Mexican Internet pharmacies will start legally selling transdermal testosterone (and estriol) creams by mail. Meanwhile you can choose to make your own from testosterone suspensions as discussed earlier.

If you take natural testosterone by mouth it will basically be broken down as it passes through the liver. If you take large amounts (i.e. 120 mg for men) orally of an ester salt like cyprionate or undecanoate only a very small percent of it will be absorbed and much unwanted toxic metabolites will be produced with serious side effects resulting.

At the University of Munster in 2002 (European Journal of Endocrinology v. 146, pp. 505-11) hypogonadal men were given 120 mg a day of oral undecanoate. This shows how poorly oral testosterone salts are absorbed to give them literally 3,000 percent (thirty times) what they need. Men only make 6 to 8 mg a day and need only 3-5 mg as a daily supplement. Of course their estrogen levels went off the scale. Even though these men were given the wrong type of testosterone in the wrong way they still got impressive benefits, albeit with side effects. If they had used natural testosterone in natural ways they would have gotten better benefits and no side effects from estrogen excess.

You can use natural sublingual testosterone in very small 3-5 mg per drop doses for men, and 0.15-0.30 milligrams (150-300 micrograms) per drop for women, but this is almost unknown. A compounding pharmacist should be able to make this upon request in a vegetable oil solution. (Testosterone does not taste good at all however.) At UCLA in Torrance in 1996 (Journal of Clinical Endocrinology and Metabolism v. 81, pp. 3654-62) hypogonadal men aged 19 to 60 were given sublingual testosterone. Unfortunately, they were given 15 mg doses, which made their testosterone go up about 500% and their estradiol almost 400 percent. At least their FSH and LH levels fell, which is usually desirable for men. Obviously the sublingual route is very effective for a mere 15 mg to put the men completely out of range like that. Even with this overdosing the men got dramatic short term benefits such as increased lean muscle mass (but not less body fat), more strength, better bone metabolism and better blood parameters. If they had given these men proper 3-5 mg doses the results would have been better and there would have been no side effects. We can still learn important lessons with such excessive doses in that sublingual route is very effective and very practical, and using low amounts will not aromatise into estradiol or estrone. The real value of this kind of hard to find study is that the sublingual route is the most effective natural legal means we have as regards actual absorption.

If you can obtain liquid testosterone in water (the usual means of injectable) you can do this yourself if you're careful. Evaporate the solution to dryness. For every gram of testosterone powder you have 333 X 3 mg, 250 X 4 mg or 200 X 5 mg doses. Just add 333, 250 or 200 drops of vegetable oil respectively and stir. Put one drop under your tongue everyday in the morning for three months and test for testosterone, estradiol and estrone. Always do this before noon to follow the natural cycle. This does not taste good. Your doctor and compounding pharmacist may or may not be willing to do this for you.

Injections of ester salts like propionate or enanthate are absolutely the worst possible means of delivery. Anyone who advises this is demonstrating their complete lack of knowledge. You will find very expensive so-called life extension doctors giving such injections because they are quacks. The problem here is that you get a huge rise in testosterone way over the normal range which falls daily until you are back to your subnormal levels by the next injection. In addition your estrone and estradiol levels increase grossly thereby exceeding your normal ranges. While patches are technically transdermal and do use natural testosterone they are very expensive, completely unnecessary and cause skin irritation from being left on day after day.

The most practical and effective means of delivery — aside from sublingual — is the transdermal route using natural, unsalted testosterone in either a cream or a gel. Again, DMSO solutions cannot be studied or used legally, but you can make your own.

Unfortunately you cannot buy a testosterone nasal spray. This would be a very effective, convenient and inexpensive way to put this right in a mucous membrane. The FDA will not allow doctors to prescribe this, pharmaceutical companies to make this, or compounding pharmacists to formulate this. If you had 99 percent USP natural testosterone you could make a 1 percent suspension (not solution) in 90 percent water with 10 percent ethanol and keep it refrigerated. Some nasal pumps deliver 100 mg of spray with each pump, so each pump would deliver 1 mg in the nasal mucosa. Three pumps therefore would deliver 3 mg most all of which would be absorbed. Researchers at the U. of Rhode Island in 1998 developed such a simple nasal delivery with excellent effectiveness but it is not approved for use even by prescription.

Again, you cannot legally buy transdermal testosterone in DMSO (dimethylsulfoxide), but you can add DMSO to your cream or gel yourself to make it more effective. If you took 100 g of 3 percent cream for men and added 100 g of DMSO you would then still use the usual quarter gram daily since it is so much more effective transdermally. A woman would add 100 g of DMSO to 100 g of 0.3 percent cream and still use the usual quarter gram. This would at least double the effectiveness of your cream or gel. DMSO is inexpensive, safe and readily available on the Internet. The very most effective natural delivery system is sublingual testosterone in DMSO solution.

Some very good work was done by SmithKline Beecham pharmaceuticals in 1996 (Journal of Clinical Pharmacology v. 36, pp.732-9). They did use expensive patches, which they referred to as "delivery systems" because that is what they produce for profit. You should understand that a year's worth of patches is only about 7 grams of testosterone at a cost of about $10. They charge over $1,300 a year for the patches so the profit margin is quite obvious. They used 2.5 mg, 5.0 mg and 7.5 mg of actually delivered testosterone in hypogonadal men aged 35-56. They did not say how many mg are contained in the Androderm® patch and what per cent of that actually went into the blood. The 2.5 mg delivered dose barely raised their levels to low normal. The 5 mg dose brought up the levels by about 50% into normal desired range. The 7.5 mg put the men unnecessarily into the high normal range This was a very thorough and well done study where they clearly distinguished between bound and bioavailable levels and compared them. They also pointed out that testosterone applied directly to the scrotum results in 5-alpha reductase activity, which converts this into high levels of undesirable DHT. The point here is that when 5 mg actually enter the bloodstream this is a practical dose to start with and will work for some men, but too high for others. Women only need 150-300 mcg (micrograms) delivered as they utilize this more efficiently than men.

SmithKline Beechum did another study in 1998 (Journal of Clinical Pharmacology v. 38, pp. 54-90). Here they just used the 5 mg delivered dose since it was the most practical and effective. Again, they used the patches on thin skin such as the back. Here they reveal that the 5 mg delivered patch contains 24.4 mg of testosterone, so only about 20 percent goes into the blood while it is applied. DHT and estradiol did not go up with such normal doses. The only drawback here is the high cost of the patches, whereas creams and gels are inexpensive.

At UCLA in Torrance in 2000 (Journal of Clinical Endocrinology and Metabolism v. 85, pp. 964-9) the researchers used a 1% gel on hypogonadal men aged 26-59 years old. The problem here is that they applied 10 grams (!) a day which is 100 mg of hormone. The blood levels went up a dangerous 500 percent and the DHT and estradiol levels also rose dangerously. What is wrong with these people? They should add a permeation enhancer to their gel since they only claimed a 10 percent delivery. Applying, say, 20 mg and delivering 5 mg into the blood would have given good results. They noted that the average male production is only 6-7 mg a day. Imagine slathering ten grams of gel on your body every day! If they had done the equivalent with women they would have used one gram of gel with 10 mg of testosterone and caused severe androgenocity. You wonder how educated people can do such things. One revelation was that it is better to use four different sites for application rather than one single site for better penetration.

These very same researchers published another study in the same journal (p. 4500-10) where they even compared the 5 mg delivered patch. They still couldn't figure out that applying 100 mg of testosterone was completely irresponsible. At least this time they did try a 5-gram gel as well as their usual 10 gram dose. They still didn't figure it out.

Incredibly these same people did a third study in the same journal (p. 2839-53) wasting fifteen more pages. In this study they cut the dose down to 5 grams of gel (50 mg of testosterone). They found that men increased lean muscle mass and strength, had better blood parameters, decreased fat mass, improved their mood, enhanced their sexual activity and generally benefited dramatically from the treatment. They claim their hydroalcoholic gel only delivers less than 12 percent of the contained testosterone, so they should find a permeation enhancer to improve poor performance.

More studies on the Androderm® patches were done at the famous Karolinska Institute in Sweden in 1997 (Clinical Endocrinology v. 47, pp. 727-37). The men aged 21-65 were given the 5 mg delivered patches and raised their testosterone immediately to desired youthful levels without raising estradiol or DHT. They also lowered FSH and LH that is a desirable benefit in aging men. The men were first subjected to testosterone enanthate injections of over 200 mg every three weeks that produced the usual terrible results. Intramuscular (i.m.) injections gave extreme peaks of 42 nmol and extreme lows of only 7 nmol (normal is about 24 nmol). The patches, on the other hand, produced excellent results with the exception of skin irritation in some men. The usual physical and psychological benefits were achieved including curing gynecomastia (male breast growth), weight loss, increased libido, less depression and improved mood.

At the well known Johns Hopkins Center in Baltimore in 2001 (Journal of Clinical Endocrinology & Metabolism, v. 86, pp. 1026-33) a more professional study was done with seventy references. The transdermal patches were used with excellent results. Hypogonadal men aged 21-65 were first given the intramuscular injections of enanthate ester. This, as usual, resulted in extreme fluctuations with over range and then under range values between the injections. This also resulted in extreme fluctuations with very high estradiol levels. The men using the patches very much improved their vital testosterone to estrogen ratios. They found that that low testosterone was correlated with a generally higher BMI (body mass index) and higher testosterone with lower BMI. Low testosterone is very correlated with obesity in other words. There were many of the usual benefits associated with raising their levels to youthful ones. Intelligent, professional studies like this using natural testosterone to produce normal levels will change medicine and demonstrate the proper use of supplemental hormones.

Other doctors walk in perpetual darkness it seems. Surprisingly, at the Karolinska Institute in 1995 (Journal of Steroid Biochemistry v. 55, pp. 121-7) healthy young men with naturally high testosterone were given weekly injections of 250 mg of testosterone enanthate. The rationale for this egregious behavior was to help determine how to detect illegal steroid use in professional athletes. Estrone and estradiol levels went through the roof and stayed there for the entire nine-month period. Testosterone went way over normal levels in these young healthy men. LH (luteinizing hormone) almost disappeared and the testosterone to LH ratio went up one thousand (i.e. 1,000) times! There is no point in wasting any more time on such complete lack of professionalism other than to demonstrate how callous some doctors can be to the very health and well being of their patients.

To show you how some doctors do not want to advance, learn, grow or improve medical practice we just have to look at a 2001 review with a full forty-three references from Massachusetts General Hospital in Boston. Here, after reviewing much of the vast body of worldwide published literature on the many proven benefits of testosterone they still call this "controversial". They were insightful enough to admit that oral and injected routes are very inferior to the transdermal delivery method as the safest and most effective means of supplementation. Yet, their conclusion was, "In summary, the potential benefit of testosterone in the aging male is still controversial and awaits the results of large, randomized, placebo-conrolled studies." They go on to say, "Testosterone therapy has the potential to cause a number of adverse events and is classi-

31

fied as a Schedule III controlled substance." There are no adverse events whatsoever when natural testosterone is used transdermally in proper amounts. Some people just hate progress obviously.

More incompetence comes from the University of Munster in 2002 (Journal of Andrology v. 23, pp. 419-25) where unfortunate men were injected with 1,000 mg (yes, that is one whole gram) of testosterone undecanoate esters every six weeks for over three years. Testosterone levels would go to dangerous heights and then fall again to subnormal levels. Estradiol levels went off the charts. They claimed "no statistically significant changes in prostate volume" occurred, but the average prostate size almost doubled due to the extreme estradiol and estrone levels. These misguided souls concluded, "injections of TU at intervals of up to three months offer an excellent alternative for substitution therapy of male hypogonadism." A mental institution might be an appropriate place for such practitioners.

A revealing study was done at Koln University in Germany in 1999 (Metabolism Clinics and Experiments v. 48, pp. 590-6). Here hypogonadal men were given four different delivery systems: 1) 100 mg oral mesterolone, 2) 160 mg oral undecanoate ester, 3) 250 mg i.m injected enanthate ester every second day, and 4) a 1,200 mg crystalline (s.c.) subcuteaneous implant. In 1999 at a major European university this is how incompetent top physicians are. Mesterolone is a dangerous, toxic anabolic steroid, and 25 mg is the normal dose. Huge oral doses of esters are toxic and raise estradiol levels. Such dangerous injections of esters every two days have severe side effects. A crystalline implant of 1,200 mg delivers far too much testosterone too quickly. After poisoning these poor men four different ways they said their total cholesterol, LDL, and triglycerides rose while HDL fell. Words fail me here.

Chapter 6: General Benefits

Almost every single study regarding the general benefits of testosterone supplementation has concerned men. A very few concerned both men and women to some degree. The little research on women and androgens has been concerned mostly with excessive hormones. "Modern day" science is so backwards that the idea of giving testosterone to women is just not comprehensible yet. "(The) last few years in the androgen field can only be described in the words of Charles Dickens, as 'the age of wisdom, (and)...the age of foolishness'." (Courtesy of Dr. Bhasin at Drew University.) Women should just realize that maintaining normal, youthful testosterone levels will give them the same basic benefits that men get. Women, like men, can test their own levels with saliva kits without using a doctor. If their level is too high they can lower it with better diet and lifestyle. If their level is too low they can raise it with very low doses of sublingual or transdermal preparations.

This chapter will be arduous to write for several reasons. There are countless studies showing the many benefits of keeping youthful testosterone levels, so the amount of information is simply overwhelming. There is also a lot of overlap with the other chapters as to specific benefits. There is just no way to clearly separate or compartmentalize these various advantages. The media and medical profession continue to tell us that testosterone replacement therapy is "unproven" and may even have "serious side effects". Any side effects are *always* due to using the wrong types in the wrong ways. This is a review of the general benefits, so there will be some repetition from other chapters. It is inexcusable that the vast majority of doctors refuse to admit the obvious and common sense benefits to raising testosterone levels in aging men and women who are deficient in this very basic hormone. The scientific literature is full of studies showing many dramatic advantages of giving testosterone to men (no women need apply!) who are deficient. Even when the wrong types and delivery systems are used - which is most all of the time - the benefits are still dramatic and impressive. Medical doctors seem to have a common mentality of overcaution and understatement, yet international studies - especially in the last ten years- clearly proclaim how adventagious testosterone supplementation is in men and women who have low levels.

It just can't be repeated too often that when men and women of any age who are testosterone deficient are given natural supplemental testosterone in natural ways there are countless benefits and no side effects whatsoever. There are *never* any side effects to supplementing low hormone levels naturally. The ideal is the youthful level you enjoyed at about the age of thirty years old. Even when the wrong forms are given in the wrong ways there are still dramatic benefits. Since at least 95 percent of the research is done using the wrong forms in the wrong ways, the best means to deal with this chapter is to concentrate on the few studies that used natural testosterone transdermally and sublingually (scientists cannot use DMSO delivery unfortunately due to the laws).

A rather amazing study was done over a half century ago (Journal of the American Medical Association v. 126, 1944, pp. 472-6) regarding the "male climacteric". Middle-aged men were given injections of testosterone salts (it was all they had at the time) and very dramatic benefits were found in only two weeks! "Definite improvement in the symptomatology was noted by the the end of the second week in all of the cases treated. Sexual potency was restored to normal with these doses (25 mg i.m. five days a week) in all but 2 (of the 29) cases." This was groundbreaking stuff six decades ago.

Dr. Alex Vermeulen at the University Hospital in Belgium is someone who has probably done more research than anyone else on hormones, yet he still doesn't understand that testosterone is *good* for prostate health and that low testosterone is a basic *cause* of prostate disease. He claims estrogen falls in men as they age (JCEM 86, 2001, pp. 2380-90) and supplemental estrogen is somehow good for men! He actually promotes estrogen therapy and androgen ablation for prostate disease! He recently did finally admit that testosterone replacement is important and men lose 60 percent of their free testosterone by the age of seventy. He also admits that supplementation is called for even with prostate enlargement. This is really something for a traditionalist like him. He should see that literally 90 percent of men over the age of fifty would benefit from supplementation. He needs to realize that *youthful* levels are the ideal and not average ranges in old age. Nevertheless, he does document the general benefits of raising testosterone in men and women as they age and is now aware of transdermal delivery.

His many published studies on testosterone and other hormones are very positive overall. His concern with "risks" is really due to using the wrong types in the wrong ways, but he can't see that. He demonstrates that testosterone is vital to bone health, sexual performance, muscle mass, strength, CHD health, cognition and memory, body mass index and body fat, blood glucose metabolism, energy levels, and feelings of well being and depression. Dr. Vermeulen even covers the various types of testosterone including injectable salts, oral salts, subcutaneous pellets, patches, gels and sublingual forms, yet he can't seem to see how dangerous and damaging the injectable and oral salts are, or how unnecessary the patches are. He did not study women when his research could be of great benefit to the women of the world.

Lisa Tenover at Emory University is the second leading researcher on hormone replacement and has published many articles on the subject. Why doesn't she include women in her various studies? Overlooking how beneficial testosterone is for both men and women, in her many reviews she always warns about the "dangers" of androgen replacement and thinks supplemental testosterone is bad for the heart and prostate. She doesn't seem to see that any "risks" are due to using the wrong types of testosterone in the wrong ways. She also can't seem to figure out that transdermal (or sublingual) dosing is the natural way to supplement hormones like testosterone, progesterone and estriol. Nevertheless, she admits there are many benefits to raising testosterone in men and women who are deficient. She feels "4 percent of men in the 40-70 year age range would be hypogonadal" when the facts are that at least 90% of men over the age of fifty are hypogonadal and would benefit greatly by raising the levels of free testosterone. She doesn't seem to see that free, not bound levels, are the only ones with any meaning. By ignoring the facts researchers are holding back science by damning testosterone with very faint praise.

Her many studies have shown great improvements in health generally with testosterone no matter which forms were used in what ways. For example, hypogonadal men were given patches to place on their scrotums, although the scrotum has high alpha reductase activity and is not a suitable place to apply testosterone (but is ideal for other hormones such as progesterone). Patches, as we have discussed, are expensive, uncomfortable and unnecessary. These men were unusual in that the average age was only 36. They were treated for at least seven years, so the long-term effects were documented. Bone density increased and their bones got stronger. This proves testosterone is vital to bone and joint health. Their prostate health was good in all facets including sonogram analysis for actual prostate volume. This proves 99.9 percent of the medical doctors in the world are wrong about their antiquated ideas on prostate health. Their testosterone to estradiol ratio improved greatly by a factor of more than 100 percent. There were no side effects at all. Finally, she saw the usual injection of unnatural esters salts don't work, never did, and never will for many reasons. Why doesn't she study women? Why doesn't she realize that natural testosterone given in natural ways is the way to go? Lisa keeps using the wrong types in the wrong ways but still gets dramatic benefits in men (why isn't she helping other women?). In one of her many published studies (Endocrine and Metabolism Clinics, v. 27, 1998, pp. 969-87) she shows men improve muscle mass, strength, body mass index, and other parameters.

If the endocrine researchers of the world would just wake up to the facts they could be guiding lights in the medical world. If they would just use natural testosterone — and all other basic hormones - in natural ways in both men and women they would find even more dramatic benefits with no side effects at all. Men and women, especially over the age of forty, would then be routinely tested for testosterone and *all* their other basic hormone levels and supplemented as needed. These doctors are fully aware that testosterone supplementation results in higher muscle mass and strength, CHD health, better mood, clearer mentality and cognition, increased libido and sexual satisfaction, better quality of life in general and all the other benefits we've discussed in this book.

Some good and heavily documented research came from such well-known institutions as Johns Hopkins University and UCLA (American Journal of Medicine v. 110, 2001, pp. 563-72, Journal of Clinical Endocrinology and Metabolism v. 82, 1997, pp. 3793-6, and Drugs and Aging v. 15, 1999, pp. 131-42). Of course, they are just concerned with men, but women will get parallel benefits in every basic way. They show oral and injected ester salts as well as implanted pellets don't work well, but newer transdermal patch systems are effective. Monitoring serum levels is emphasized to insure safety and effectiveness. They realize that testosterone does not cause nor worsen prostate cancer to their credit. Body composition, lean muscle mass, physical strength and body fat are all improved by testosterone therapy. Sexual functioning and genital dysfunction (such as low sperm count and small penis) are improved, but this is no panacea for impotence. They found that many diseases are correlated with low levels of testosterone such as HIV and coronary heart conditions. "There is a substantial prevalence of low testosterone levels in men with cancer." Psychology is improved especially cognition, mood, depression, memory and sense of well being with testosterone supplementation. "Many autoimmune diseases are associated with low testosterone levels." Bones are stronger with youthful testosterone levels. "Reversal of hypogonadism is associated with improvement in bone mass and maintenance of skeletal integrity." Blood parameters such as anemia, hemocrit and hemoglobin values are improved with supplementary testosterone as well. All in all, they see that as men get older their testosterone levels fall and are clearly correlated with every problem of aging. They do point out that women only produce about 150 mcg of testosterone from their ovaries after menopause. Women with hysterectomies (one third of American women) are generally testosterone deficient. Women may get many other benefits from testosterone supplementation after menopause, but more research is needed. Why aren't these researchers doing this much-needed research on women? They are clearly in favor of routine androgen therapy in men as they age. Soon such clinicians are going to be making the same recommendations for women.

At Christie Hospital in England men were given 5 mg a day of testosterone via patches (Hormone Research v. 56, 2000, pp. 86-92). The subjects had improved body composition, lean mass and less body fat. Their psychology improved overall. Sexual function was much better. Bone density was higher. Cardiovascular health was better. They were still concerned with prostate cancer because they don't yet understand that youthful levels of testosterone are necessary for good prostate health. There were sixty references to other studies showing the validity of testosterone supplementation in aging men.

At Harbor University in Los Angeles (Journal of Clinical Endocrinology and Metabolism v.85, 2000, pp. 2839-53) transdermal gel was used delivering 10 mg a day to men. This sounds low, but it is still too much considering men only produce 6-8 mg a day and 3-5 mg is a much safer dose. "We conclude that testosterone gel replacement improved sexual function and mood, increased lean mass and muscle strength and decreased fat mass in hypogonadal men with less skin irritation and discontinuation compared with the recommended dose of the permeating-enhanced testosterone patch." This was a long fifteen page study with a full forty-five references.

This chapter on general benefits could easily take up the entire book. We have only chosen a few of the countless studies to show there is no doubt about the need for supplementary testosterone in men and women who are low, regardless of their age. In the last five years there have finally been studies on testosterone therapy for women and this will continue to increase.

Chapter 7: Cardiovascular Health

The biggest killer of Americans by far - especially men - is cardiovascular disease (CHD). Therefore an entire chapter will be devoted to CHD conditions. The vast majority of the medical profession still lives in the Dark Ages here and feels that men suffer from more CHD because they have much higher testosterone levels than women! There is overwhelming evidence to show that men with higher testosterone levels have much healthier hearts and circulatory systems with longer and better quality of life. We badly need similar studies in women, but current research, common sense and logic tell us that women with normal, youthful testosterone levels have the same protective benefits (women with hyper levels of testosterone, on the other hand, suffer from more cardiovascular problems). Ideally we would concentrate on supplemental studies using transdermal (or sublingual) delivery, but such studies are very hard to find concerning heart and artery health.

The most impressive review was fourteen pages from the Danish Center for Clinical Research in 1996 (Atherosclerosis, v. 125, p. 1-13) with a comprehensive analysis of eighty-five studies. Such a lengthy review leaves no doubt about testosterone being a heart healthy hormone. "In conclusion, one intervention, eight cohort and several (there were 30) cross-sectional studies suggest either a neutral or a favorable effect of testosterone and DHEA(S) on CHD in males."

The largest cross-sectional study in 1987 of 2,512 men (American Journal of Epidemiology, v. 126, pp. 647-57) concluded, "Subjects with prevalent ischemic heart disease were reported to have significantly lower serum testosterone levels than subjects without IHD." That one sentence says it all.

The University of Sheffield in England did more studies in this area than any other institution. In 2000 (European Heart Journal, v. 21, pp. 890-4) ninety men were studied. They concluded,

"Men with coronary artery heart disease have significantly lower levels of androgens than normal controls, challenging the preconception that physiologically high levels of androgens in men account for their increased relative risk for coronary heart artery disease." They exposed the unsubstantiated myth that testosterone is somehow bad for men — a myth which is still very prevalent today in the medical profession. They further said, "High androgen levels are presumed by many to explain the male predisposition to coronary artery disease. However, natural androgens inhibit male atherosclerosis." Further, "There is also increasing evidence in the literature to show that low levels of androgens are associated with adverse cardiovascular risk factors including an atherogenic lipid profile, systolic and diastolic hypertension, obesity, insulin resistance, and raised fibrinogen in humans." Free testosterone levels were emphatically emphasized, *"This study shows that there is a positive associate between low serum androgen levels and the presence of coronary artery disease."* The heart patients also had high levels of LH and FSH. This is exemplary science! In the same journal (v. 24, 2003, pp. 909-15) they further said, "Administration of testosterone increases cardiac output acutely."

In the same year at this university (Circulation, v. 102, pp. 1906-11) some more very smart doctors gave transdermal 5 mg (delivered) testosterone patches for three months to elderly men who suffered from chronic angina (heart inflammation) in a double blind study. The free testosterone levels rose from 46-73 (59%) on the average and their LH and FSH fell dramatically (which is good for men). Their estrogen levels did not rise. "Low dose supplemental testosterone treatment in men with chronic stable angina reduces exercise-induced myocardial ischemia (blocked arterial flow)." This means the men on testosterone could now exercise more freely. Aside from the cardiac benefits, these men improved greatly in general physical functioning, social functioning, mental health, overall vitality, freedom from pain and general perception of their health.

A fourth study there (Quarterly Journal of Medicine, v. 90, 1997, pp. 787-91) was a review of the literature. They showed that,

"Low mean levels of testosterone have been found in populations of hypertensive men. In men, high levels of estrogen and estrone are associated with increased risks of myocardial infarction, angina, and CAD. Estrogens given to male survivors of myocardial infarction lead to an increased re-infarction rate. Giving estrogens to men with prostatic carcinoma is associated with increased mortality from CAD (coronary artery disease)." It is obvious that testosterone, androstenedione and DHEA are heart protective, while excess estradiol and estrone cause heart disease. Yet a fifth study there (Heart, v. 89, 2003, pp. 121-2) found, "…administration of low physiologic replacement doses of testosterone over three months in men with chronic stable angina significantly improves exercise tolerance and angina threshold."

From Imperial College in London in 1999 (American Journal of Cardiology, v. 83, pp. 437-9), men aged 35-75, were given intravenous infusions of 2.3 mg of natural testosterone. All of them were suffering from angina, so relaxing their arteries was very beneficial. They found the majority of these men to be testosterone deficient. Giving them the infusions, "increases time to onset of exercise-induced myocardial ischemia in men with CAD who have decreased plasma testosterone." In plain English this means the supplemental testosterone improved the arterial constrictions during exercise and allowed more blood flow. They quoted twenty-two other studies showing the general benefits of testosterone supplementation for improved heart and artery health. Another study (Circulation v. 99, 1999, pp. 1666-70) from the San Raffaele Institute in Italy confirmed these same facts. "Short-term administration of testosterone induces a beneficial effect on exercise-induced myocardial ischemia in men with coronary heart disease." What could be clearer?

One of the few studies that included women was from University Hospital in Belgium in 1996 (Sex Steroids Cardiovascular Systems 1st, pp. 181-200). Women can naturally suffer from excessive testosterone levels while men cannot. Women who have such hyper levels do suffer from more heart and artery conditions, but youthful levels in women were correlated with less CHD problems.

They went on to also discuss the beneficial effects of normal testosterone levels on insulin function in both men and women. We need a lot more work like this regarding women.

At the INSERM research facility in France the Telecom Study was done in 1997 (Journal of Clinical Endocrinology and Metabolism, v. 82, pp. 682-5). They found, "Compared to the men with higher testosterone, the men with low testosterone had a significantly higher body mass index, higher waist/hip ratio, higher systolic blood pressure, and higher fasting and 2-hour plasma insulin." Here they saw an important inverse relationship where the higher the testosterone level, the lower the insulin level. Hyperinsulemia and insulin resistance with excessive insulin levels are epidemic in Western societies in both men and women, so lowering insulin levels generally is very positive.

At the Hunan University in China in 1998 (Hunan Yike Daxue Xuebao, v. 23, p. 299-301) healthy men were compared to men with coronary heart disease and studied for their sex hormone levels as related to their blood lipids. Here the doctors found that the higher the testosterone the higher the "good" HDL cholesterol and the lower the triglycerides. They concluded, "The results suggest that the endogenous testosterone in males regulates the blood lipid metabolism, and the male with low plasma testosterone might be lead to blood lipid metabolism abnormality, is a risk factor of coronary disease." Youthful testosterone levels help keep blood fats low.

Another Chinese study from the Tongji Medical University in 1998 (Zhongguo Bingli Shengli Zazhi, v. 14, pp. 745-7) found that men with low testosterone and low HDL cholesterol and high estrogen-to-testosterone ratios (too much estrogen and too little testosterone) were more prone to CHD problems. They also showed that the higher the testosterone the higher the HDL ("good") cholesterol levels. They concluded, "The imbalance of sex hormones mainly induced by the decrease of testosterone level was a pathogenic factor for CHD in the male." Well stated.

When it comes to cholesterol and blood lipids the literature on supplemental testosterone seems to be conflicting. Some studies on testosterone therapy show better total cholesterol, HDL, LDL, and triglyceride levels, while others show no benefits. The reason is that when the wrong forms are given in the wrong ways blood lipids are usually not improved. When transdermal natural testosterone is used there are always improvements in blood fats.

At Bielanski Hospital in Poland in 1996 (Atherosclerosis, v. 121, pp. 35-43) men with low testosterone were given 200 mg i.m. injections of enanthate ester every second week for a year. Total cholesterol fell from an average of 225-198 mg and LDL 139-118 mg with no change in diet. Even giving these men the wrong kind of testosterone in the wrong way resulted in dramatic improvement in their blood lipids. "The results of this study indicate that testosterone replacement therapy in hypogonadal and elderly men may have a beneficial effect on lipid metabolism through decreasing total cholesterol and atherogenic fraction of LDL cholesterol."

Similar results were found at the University of Texas in San Antonio in 1993 (Journal of Clinical Endocrinology and Metabolism, v. 77, p. 1610-15). The researchers said, "In conclusion the authors observed a less atherogenic lipid and lipoprotein profile with increased testosterone concentrations." This included DHEA as well. At the same university in 1996 (Journal of Clinical Endocrinology and Metabolism v. 81, pp. 3697-3701) some of the same researchers found that low testosterone levels in men equated clearly with high LDL ("bad") levels. "In conclusion, we have shown that men with decreased concentrations of total testosterone and SHBG have an unfavorable composition of LDL." They refer to other studies that found low testosterone is also associated with lower HDL levels and higher triglyceride levels.

We could go on with dozens and dozens of studies like this. To name a few more: At Vrije University in the Netherlands (Aging Male, v. 4, 2001, pp. 30-8) the evidence clearly showed, "Epidemiological studies show, however, that men with cardiovascular disease have low rather than high circulating testosterone." At the University of Bari in Italy (Metabolism & Clinical Experiments, v. 45, 1997, pp. 1289-93) a very in-depth and complex study was done on multiple cardiovascular factors. They concluded, "Thus, because of the increase of several prothrombic factors, men with central obesity, particularly those with lower androgenicity, seem to be at greater risk for CHD." At Royal Brompton Hospital in London testosterone was given to men with CHD. "Short term intracoronary administration of testosterone at physiological concentrations, induces coronary artery dilation and increases coronary blood flow in men with established CHD."

Heart disease in women was studied over a five year period in Chile (Maturitas, v. 45, 2003, pp. 205-12). Women 40 to 59 were evaluated and then re-evaluated five years later. The risk factors were found to be sedentarism (laying on their dead rear ends), high cholesterol and triglycerides, hypertension, obesity, smoking and diabetes. Hormone levels were not measured in this otherwise excellent study, however.

Testosterone deficiency and female cardiovascular disease were covered in a very rare report published in the Journal of Women's Health in 1998 (v. 7, pp. 825-9). "Restoring a physiologic level of testosterone-to-women after hysterectomy not only can improve quality of life in terms of sexual libido, sexual pleasure, and sense of well-being, but also can build bones — and may be a key to protecting cardiovascular health. Women developing testosterone deficiency as a consequence of natural aging/menopause may similarly benefit from physiologic testosterone supplementation." There is no doubt that youthful testosterone levels in men supports heart health. When we do more studies on women we'll find the same situation. Women must be careful to maintain normal range levels, as excessive androgens are just as harmful as deficient ones. Youthful levels of androgens (including androstenedione and DHEA) for both men and women are vital to good cardiovascular health and long life.

Chapter 8: Various Diseases and Testosterone

The proper way to cure any disease, illness or condition is with natural diet, proven supplements, balancing your basic hormones, fasting, exercise, and avoiding negative habits (like coffee, alcohol, etc.). Total natural lifestyle in other words. Please read my book *Zen Macrobiotics for Americans* to learn more about this. Few conditions have been studied for their relation to testosterone levels. What little work has been done is still almost unknown to the medical profession, much less to the general public, and remain hidden in medical journals. We very much need more research on how testosterone levels affect common illnesses especially regarding women. In going back twenty years on such research as listed in Chemical Abstracts very, very little was found. As always, all our hormones work together in harmony as a team, and this endocrine "concert" is vital to every aspect of our health and wellbeing. Testosterone is only one of our dozen basic hormones that need to be measured and balanced (see Chapter 17 for more on this). Supplemental testosterone is very limited in effect if various other hormones are out of balance. While there is a paucity of published studies on how testosterone levels affect various diseases, the ones we have clearly demonstrate just how important our levels are for good health. We always have to keep in mind that men can only suffer from low testosterone, while women can suffer from both hypo- and hyper- levels.

The best study of all was "Androgen Therapy in Non-endocrine Illnesses" (Androgens and Androgen Receptors, pub. 2002) from Vermont University with 23 pages and 132 references. This concentrated on critical illness in general, AIDS, renal failure and pulmonary disease. Due to the overall anabolic effects of testosterone it is suggested that any illness where the person is proven to be testosterone deficient may benefit from supplementation. This is excellent, progressive, and well-documented work covering a wide range of conditions.

Fortunately there has been some good work done concerning AIDS in both men and women. The fact this very devastating and incurable disease can be dramatically benefited by testosterone therapy shows us great promise in other illnesses. AIDS is not curable by natural means because it is a product of the biowarfare research laboratories; it is a genetically engineered virus unknown to nature. Restoring youthful testosterone levels has yielded rather impressive benefits for people suffering from AIDS. At Massachusetts General Hospital (Archives of Internal Medicine, v. 164, pp. 897-904) women with AIDS were given testosterone patches with striking results. "We found that giving natural testosterone at levels that are normal for women produces significant improvement for patients with few other treatment options." Again, at this hospital (Journal of Clinical Endocrinology & Metabolism, v. 83, 1998, pp. 2717-25) more women with AIDS with proven deficiency were given testosterone patches. Very dramatic improvement was noted with no other treatment. At Harvard Medical School (Journal of Clinical Endocrinology & Metabolism, v. 83, 1998, pp. 2717-25) the same results were found for women using 150 to 300 mcg daily. At the New York State Psychiatric Institute men with AIDS responded well to testosterone supplementation. At Drew University male AIDS patients aged 18-60 were given natural transdermal patches with powerful results. At the famous Johns Hopkins University in Baltimore men with AIDS were given supplemental testosterone. "Hypogonadal men who are given testosterone replacement have improved sexual thoughts and functioning, more energy and improved mood." Generally, quality of life improves with such therapy.

At the Gujaret Cancer Society in India (Neoplasma, v. 41, 1994) male (why not women?) lung cancer patients were studied for a wide range of twelve hormone and other diagnostic factors. This was a very impressive and comprehensive study. The advanced cancer patients had 32 percent less testosterone as well as 47 percent less DHEA. They also had 23 percent lower progesterone (it is rare to test men for progesterone) levels, but 17 percent higher estradiol levels. It is rare and groundbreaking research such as this that shows us how hormones affect disease states. We need much more similar research done in this area.

Diabetes is a growing epidemic in America especially among children, Latins and Africans. At New England Research Institutes (Diabetes Care, v. 23, 2000, pp. 490-4) 1,156 men aged 40-70 were studied for ten years. "Our prospective findings are consistent with previous, mainly cross-sectional reports, suggesting that low levels of testosterone play some role in the development of insulin resistance and subsequent Type 2 diabetes."

For once women were included in studies at Erasmus Medical Center in the Netherlands (Journal of Clinical Endocrinolgy and Metabolism, v. 87, 2002, pp. 3632-9). The famous Rotterdam Study of 1,032 men and women was most comprehensive in many ways. "In conclusion, we found an independent inverse association between levels of testosterone and aortic atherosclerosis in men. In women, positive associations between levels of testosterone and aortic atherosclerosis were largely due to adverse cardiovascular disease risk factors." Here, hypertestosterone levels in women were correlated with CHD conditions, but not normal levels. In other words, youthful testosterone levels are good for women.

At Affiliated Hospital in China men with renal failure were studied (Hubei Yike Daxue Xuebao, v. 18, 1997, pp. 244-5) for their hormone levels. "Testosterone levels in patients with CRF (chronic renal failure) were significantly decreased compared with the controls." Why aren't urologists using testosterone therapy with male and female patients with kidney failure and kidney disease of all kinds?

Here are some brief specific examples of various diseases: At the University of Padova in Italy women with liver cirrhosis had low testosterone as compared to healthy controls. Both men and women with lupus (LE) were found to be testosterone deficent at the University of Mississippi. Men with liver cancer had lower testosterone levels compared to controls at Harvard Medical

School. At the University of Texas men with diabetes and insulin resistance were low in testosterone. The same thing was found at Malmo University in Sweden. Young men with Klinefelters Syndrome were treated with testosterone at Arhus Hospital in Denmark with remarkable progress for three years. At the famous Karolinska Institute in Sweden men with rheumatoid arthritis tested much lower in testosterone than healthy men of the same age. At Beth Israel Center in Boston epileptic men had impaired testosterone production and elevated estradiol levels. Men and women with stomach and colorectal cancer generally had low testosterone levels when studied at Provincial Hospital in China. At Pochon University in Korea a group of healthy men had much higher testosterone than a similar group of men suffering from various pathological conditions. Men with gout had low testosterone levels at Donetsk University in Russia.

Alzheimer's is almost an epidemic and we have almost no understanding of its cause, much less any clue as to curing it. At the University of Texas (Aging Male, v. 6, 2003, pp. 13-17) men with Alzheimer's were given testosterone injections in a double blind study. "…testosterone could indeed improve cognition, including visual-spatial skills in mild to moderate Alzheimer's disease". You didn't hear that on the six o' clock news. The same results were found at the University of Western Australia (Medical Hypotheses, v. 60, 2003, pp. 893-6) including women.

The Tromso Study in Norway (European Journal of Endocrinology v. 149, 2003, pp. 145-52) studied chronic disease in men. "Men who reported having had a stroke or cancer diagnosis had significantly lower levels of total and free testosterone." They also found the lower the testosterone level the higher the BMI (i.e. low testosterone equals obesity basically). Women were included in the Tromso Study, but strangely enough not in this review.

Regardless of what condition or illness you may or may not have you want to keep all your basic hormones at youthful levels to maintain a long, healthy life. This is covered in detail in Chapter 17 "Your Other Hormones".

Chapter 9: Osteoporosis and Bone Health

Osteoporosis is all too common and affects far more women than men. In Western societies about half of women over the age of sixty-five have serious bone loss. About one in six men of the same age also have serious bone loss. There are *no* effective medical treatments for this despite the constant onslaught of advertising to the contrary. HRT for women, for example, did not improve bone health at all. None of the heavily promoted drugs improve bone density despite the alluring claims. Ironically, poor Third World countries have far less problems with their bone and joint health. All bone and joint conditions have the same basic causes and the same basic treatments. Whether we are talking about bone loss, arthritis or tooth decay, it is basically the same metabolism at work and the same cures - diet, supplements, hormones and exercise. The only real cures are natural ones. Please read *Zen Macrobiotics for Americans* and *No More Horse Estrogen!* for more information. Finally, we have a wealth of studies on women and most of the studies in this chapter will therefore be on women. Even though bone loss affects mostly women, the majority of published studies still concerned men only! This kind of bias has to stop.

Testosterone, DHEA and androstenedione (as is progesterone) are all vital for bone growth. As we age it is important to maintain youthful DHEA (as well as progesterone) levels as well as testosterone levels to prevent bone loss in both sexes. There are many published studies fortunately showing that androgens in general are vital for bone growth, maintenance and the prevention of joint inflammation and deterioration.

Pre-, peri- and postmenopausal women were studied at Keio University in Japan in 1998 (Environmental Health and Preventive Medicine, v. 3, pp.123-9). Their clear conclusion was that "Testosterone was positively correlated with BMD (bone mineral density)." They further went on to say, "These finding suggest that endogenous androgens may exert positive influences on BMD."

Hypogonadal men with osteoporosis aged 34 to 73 were given supplemental testosterone at Freeman Hospital in the U.K (Bone, v. 18, 1996, pp. 171-7). Injections of salts every two weeks raised their levels over 50 percent and they got excellent results. "All bone markers decreased indicating that treatment suppressed bone turnover." They said further, "Thus, testosterone is a promising treatment for men with idiopathic osteoporosis, acting to suppress bone resorption." The fact that men in their thirties were already suffering from serious bone loss is rather unsettling. Even using the wrong type of testosterone in the wrong way gave dramatic results in only six months considering the fact that long (trabeculuar) bones grow slowly.

Young men were tested at the University of Lodz in Poland in 2000 (Neuroendocrine Letters, v. 21, p. 25-30) for their bone mineral density as compared to their testosterone level. The conclusion was, "There was a positive correlation between testosterone concentrations and BMD as well as T-score both in healthy subjects and in infertile patients. Results of the present study indicate that attention should be paid to testosterone deficiency in the young age in terms of the potential risk of decreased bone mineral density in the advanced age."

At Hunan University in China (Journal of Environmental Pathology, v. 19, 2000, pp. 167-9) both pre- and postmenopausal healthy women were studied. They concluded, "The bone mineral density of the lumbar spine, hip and forearm were significantly correlated with estriol and total testosterone respectively. Therefore different hormones should be considered in hormone replacement therapy." They postulated that a major reason men have stronger bones is due to their higher testosterone level.

At Indiana State University (Journal of Clincal Investigation, v. 97, 1996, pp. 14-21) 231 healthy women varying in age from 32-77 were studied for bone loss. "Bone loss was signi-

ficantly associated with lower androgen (testosterone, androstenedione and DHEA) concentrations in premenopausal women,
and with lower androgens in peri- and postmenopausal women."
Sex steroids are important for the maintenance of skeletal integrity
before menopause and for as long as 20-25 years afterwards. "Testosterone, androstenedione and DHEA all fell dramatically as the
women aged." They also found that progesterone fell a full 59 percent on the average, which also was a major factor in cases of osteoporosis.

A multi-center study headed by Emory University in At-
lanta (Journal of Clinical Endocrinology and Metabolism, v. 69,
1989, pp. 533-9) did a long five-year study for both pre- and peri-
menopausal women. Free testosterone correlated positively with
bone density, even after controlling for weight. "These data suggest that women who are still menstruating may have relative defi-
ciencies in testosterone with reduced bone densities as a consequence. We found that free testosterone correlated positively and
significantly with bone density. In summary these data highlight
the importance of testosterone in women's skeletal integrity and
stress the critical influence of hormonal factors on bone loss."

At the VA Hospital in St. Louis (Journal of Clinical Endocrinology and Metabolism, v. 81, 1996, pp. 1108-17) a combina-
tion of white and black women aged 20-90 were studied for their
bone health. Bone density declined in all women over the age of
forty although black women had slightly stronger bones, mostly
due to their having higher testosterone levels. Most were overweight (obesity has one advantage in that obese people tend to
have stronger bones in order to support their excess weight). It was
found that testosterone, DHEA and vitamin D levels were all very
important determinants of bone strength in both races and all three
fell as the women aged. This study covered women of two races
and all ages.

A double blind study at Washington University in St. Louis
(Clinical Endocrinology, v. 53, 2000, pp. 561-8) included elderly
men and women with an average age of seventy-three years. They

gave them all 50 mg of DHEA for six months. This is a very high dose for men and a completely irresponsible dose for women. Because of the overdose the men raised their testosterone 46 percent on the average and women 214 percent. Their lean muscle increased, their body fat decreased, and their bones got stronger. It should be emphasized that testosterone levels *cannot* be raised by giving normal doses of DHEA, and this happened only because these poor old people were given far too much. Doing this for a longer term would have resulted in serious side effects from hyper DHEA levels.

At the Tokyo Geriatric center in Japan in Pullman (Endocrinology Japan, v. 38, 1991, pp. 343-9) elderly postmenopausal women had many of their hormones measured along with their BMI (body mass index). The women with the highest levels of calcitonin, DHEA, androstenedione and testosterone had the strongest bones and the least fractures. Androstenedione was shown to be highly correlated with bone density at Cuore University in Rome (Experimental and Clinical Endocrinological Diabetes v. 104, 1996, 363-70). "Plasma androstenedione was the only other variable (besides PTH or para-thyroid) that contributed to spine BMI." Testosterone and DHEA were not measured here but would have made the results a lot more complete.

At the Long Island Medical Center in New York (International Journal of Gynecology and Obstetrics, v. 25, 1987, pp. 217-22) postmenopausal women were studied for DHEA and androstenedione (testosterone was not studied here). "Our data clearly indicate a positive correlation of at least two androgens with bone density." They found no such correlation for estrone or estradiol. Again, we see androgens are the bone building hormones. If testosterone had been tested they would have gotten the same results as nearly everyone else.

The above studies clearly prove the point. Androgens, especially testosterone are the bone-building hormones and both men and women should keep their testosterone levels youthful as one part of a program of total bone health.

Chapter 10: Testosterone and Your Prostate

The medical profession has an unquestioned "Huggins" dogma that testosterone is somehow "bad" for the male prostate gland. When prostate cancer patients are castrated they very temporarily (emphasis on the temporary part) improve, but their cancer then grows with a vengeance. This is Sacred Dogma, and anyone who questions it is condemned as a heretic or worse. Common sense tells you *nothing* gets better when you cut a man's testicles off - whether you use a scalpel or prescription drugs like Lupron® and Casodex®. Doctors still literally castrate men physically believe it or not. Talk about the Dark Ages!

You can see clearly from the Male Estrogen and Testosterone Chart (pp. 58) that, as men age, their estrogen rises while their testosterone falls. Young men with naturally high testosterone (and low estrogen) levels are almost completely immune to prostate disease. The fall in testosterone and rise is estrogen - the reversal of the testosterone to estrogen ratio — almost exactly parallels the rise in prostate disease of all kinds. As testosterone falls, BPH, prostatitis and prostate cancer all rise accordingly. The more youthful the testosterone level the healthier men will be in all ways.

The worldwide published clinical studies on testosterone levels and prostate health prove unequivocally beyond any doubt whatsoever that testosterone is necessary for good prostate health and metabolism. The higher the testosterone levels the lower the rates of prostate disease. The lower the testosterone levels the higher the rates of prostate disease. When men are low in testosterone the prostate receptors must accept dihydrotestosterone (DHT) instead of the real thing. Studies show that prostate disease is largely due to the gland having an inordinate amount of DHT bound to it rather than real testosterone. Youthful levels of all the androgens including DHEA and androstenedione are important to good prostate health. We are going to list a *partial* (18 out of 70)

53

and very abbreviated condensation of the chapter "Testosterone Is Your Friend" from my book *The Natural Prostate Cure*. Please see the book for all seventy of the complete studies.

All the way back in 1936 at Oxford University in England (Proceedings of the Royal Society of Medicine) doctors realized that the "male hormone" was necessary for good prostate health and the "female hormone" was bad for prostate health. Testosterone had only first been synthesized in 1935, a year earlier.

Almost seventy years ago in 1938 doctors at Louisiana State University (Journal of Urology) also knew that testosterone is good for prostate health. They realized how vital this hormone is, and that male health suffered as their levels fell during normal aging. They saw great promise in supplemental testosterone now that it was synthesized and could be given to aging men.

At the University of Washington (Cancer Research, v. 59, 1999, pp.4161-4) a progressive, innovative and free thinking doctor named Richmond Prehn actually said that we should consider giving androgen *supplements* to reduce the growth of prostate cancer! You don't know how much courage it took to say that, or for the journal *Cancer Research* to print it. He showed that earlier studies proved low testosterone levels led to a far worse prognosis than in men with higher testosterone levels. Doctors like this are leading us into the Age of Enlightenment.

At the University of Witwaterstrand in South Africa (American Journal of Clinical Oncology, v. 20, 1997, pp. 605-8) 122 men with prostate cancer were studied for their testosterone levels, "Low Serum Testosterone Predicts a Poor Outcome in Metastatic Prostate Cancer". The men with the highest levels of testosterone had the least aggressive tumors and lived the longest. The men with the lowest levels had the most aggressive tumors and died quickly. They concluded, "Low testosterone seems to result in a more aggressive disease and a poorer prognosis in advanced prostate cancer."

At Hubei Medical University in China (Hubei Yike Daxue Xeubao, v. 19, 1998, pp. 241-2) doctors studied men with BPH and outright prostate cancer. They found, "The results showed that serum testosterone in patients with BPH and PCA (cancer) was lower than that of the (healthy) control group." They said further, "...the ratio of testosterone to estradiol is decreased with the rise of the age. The results suggested that the imbalance of serum sex hormones (i.e. falling testosterone and rising estrogen) was related to the pathogenesis of BPH and PCA." This is pretty clear here, too.

At the world famous Harvard Medical School (Journal of Urology, v. 163, 2000, pp. 824-7) "Is Low Serum Testosterone a Marker for High Grade Prostate Cancer?" was published. Men with low testosterone levels had faster growing tumors, higher Gleason scores and died earlier. The conclusion was, "In our study patents with prostate cancer and a low free testosterone had more extensive disease. In addition, all men with a biopsy Gleason score of 8 or greater had low serum free testosterone. This finding suggests that low serum free testosterone may be a marker for more aggressive disease."

At the University of Vienna (Prostate, v. 44, 2000, pp. 219-24) men with prostate cancer were compared to healthy controls. The men with cancer had decidedly lower testosterone levels than their healthy counterparts. Again we see the lower the testosterone the worse the diseases rates. They also found that youthful levels of the androgen DHEA was also necessary for good prostate health.

A second study at the University of Vienna (Journal of Urology, v. 169, 2003, pp. 1312-5) also studied men with prostate cancer. "Low serum testosterone in men with newly diagnosed prostate cancer is associated with higher tumor microvessels and androgen density (both of these factors promote cancer growth) as well as higher Gleason scores suggesting enhanced malignant potential." As always, testosterone proves to be prostate healthy.

A third study at the same university (Prostate, v. 47, 2001, pp. 52-8) found the same results with more patients. This was titled, "High Grade Prostate Cancer is Associated with Low Serum Testosterone Levels". The title says it all. The men with low levels averaging only 2.8 ng/ml had the fastest growing malignancies and died faster. The men with high levels averaging 4.1 ng/ml had the slowest growing malignancies and lived the longest. Why aren't we using testosterone *supplements* for prostate cancer?

At Harvard Medical School again (Journal of the American Medical Association v. 276, 1996, pp. 1904-6) prostate cancer patients fared better and lived longer the higher their testosterone level was. "A high prevalence of biopsy-detectable prostate cancer was identified in men with low total and free testosterone." This is right from Harvard Medical School again folks. When will doctors start *treating* prostate disease with supplemental testosterone?

At the Memphis Veterans hospital (Journal of Urology, v. 144, 1989, pp. 1139-42) the military doctors found the elderly veterans with prostate cancer did much better the higher their testosterone levels. "Patients with a pretreatment level of testosterone less than 300 ng/ml had shorter intervals free of progression than patients with pretreatment levels greater than 300 ng/ml." They referred to earlier studies that found exactly the same phenomenon. Testosterone should be used as *therapy* for prostate cancer.

A review done collectively by six international clinics (Cancer, Epidemiology, Biomarkers Preview, v. 6, 1997, pp. 967-9) used the Norwegian Cancer Registry to study the frozen blood serum and medical records of over 28,000 men. They found the higher the testosterone level the less prostate cancer and the longer their life. They concluded that the popular idea that testosterone promotes prostate cancer in any way is completely unsupported by the research. This is the second largest prostate cancer study in history and the results are simply inarguable based on <u>28,000 men.</u>

At the University of Chicago and three other clinics (Journal of the American Medical Association, v. 265, 1991, pp. 618-

21) more men with prostate cancer were studied. Divided into four groups of low to high testosterone each group clearly progressively thrived as their testosterone rating rose. The lowest group did the worst, while the highest group had the best quality of life, lived the longest, and their cancer grew the slowest.

At the famous Johns Hopkins Center in Baltimore (Prostate v. 27, 1995, pp. 25-31) healthy men were compared to those with BHP and prostate cancer. The healthy men had testosterone levels of 636 ng/ml, the men with BPH had 527, and the cancer patients only 473. The healthy men had full one-third higher testosterone levels than cancer patients — a very dramatic difference. Yet the doctors tried to deny their own data since it didn't fit into their bias! "These data suggest there are no measurable differences in serum testosterone levels among men who are destined to develop prostate cancer and those without the disease"! How can there be "no measurable differences" between levels of 636 ng in healthy men and only 473 ng in cancer patients? This is the kind of blindness that keeps the medical profession perpetually in the dark.

At the University of Utah (Journal of Clinical Endocrinology and Metabolism, v. 82, 1997, pp. 571-5) a very unusual study was done with 214 pairs of identical twins. Such rare studies are exceedingly accurate due to biological equality of the twins. They found the higher the testosterone the smaller the prostate glands, and the lower the testosterone the larger the prostate glands. "Prostate volume correlated inversely with age adjusted serum testosterone level." This is inarguable proof youthful and higher testosterone levels promote good prostate health and help prevent disease.

At the Petrov Institute in Russia (International Journal of Andrology, v. 25, 2002, pp. 119-25) hypogonadal men averaging only 40 years old were given 80 or 120 mg of oral testosterone undecanoate salts depending on how low their testosterone was. After only six months their prostate volumes fell. They actually shrank their prostates giving them the wrong kind of testosterone in the wrong way. Imagine how much better they would have done with low doses of sublingual or transdermal testosterone. "These data suggest that exogenous testosterone in middle aged and older men with some clinical features of age-related testosterone deficiency can retard or even reverse prostate growth."

At the Tenovus Institute in Wales (European Journal of Cancer, v. 20, 1984, pp. 477-82) 222 men with prostate cancer were studied. As usual they found the men with the lowest testosterone levels had the poorest prognosis and the earliest deaths. "Low concentrations of testosterone in plasma at the time of diagnosis related to a poor prognosis. Patients who died within one year of diagnosis had the lowest mean plasma levels of this steroid." This study was done almost twenty years ago, yet doctors continue to castrate men both chemically and surgically.

The doctors at the University of Connecticut (Endocrine Research, v.26, 2000, pp. 153-68) gave elderly men both transdermal patches and unnatural injections of salts. Nearly all American men over seventy have prostate cancer even though most of them won't actually die from it. Even giving them the wrong kind of testosterone in the wrong way did not cause any ill effects on prostate size, symptoms, or prostate specific antigen (PSA) level. "No significant side effects in prostate tests or symptoms were seen in this study." They should have diagnosed them for the many other benefits of testosterone therapy.

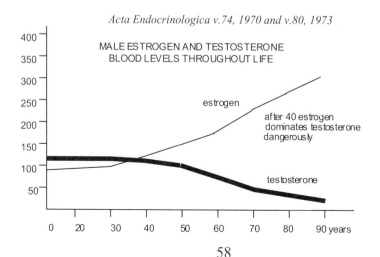

Acta Endocrinologica v.74, 1970 and v.80, 1973

MALE ESTROGEN AND TESTOSTERONE
BLOOD LEVELS THROUGHOUT LIFE

estrogen

after 40 estrogen dominates testosterone dangerously

testosterone

Chapter 11: Female Sexuality

Women looking towards using testosterone as the Magic Answer to their sexual concerns are looking in the wrong place. Sexuality for women is a multifactoral, and very emotional affair with far more psychology than biology. Female sexuality is such a complex and multifaceted phenomena that no amount of hormones could be the single answer to dysfunction. Good sex is a reflection of total physical, mental and emotional health, and not just youthful hormone levels, important as that is. Youthful testosterone levels are not even required for sexual desire as demonstrated by pre-pubertal girls, postmenopausal women and those who have had hysterectomies. Some women with low testosterone levels have very rewarding sex lives. Yes, some women are testosterone deficient, but still have satisfying sex lives.

Having said all that, we find that men are not as hormonally affected as women are either physically or psychologically. While many male studies will only show a 10 percent improvement in male sexual performance in hypogonadal men who receive testosterone supplements, you see far more dramatic improvement in women who are testosterone deficient. Women are simply more hormonally driven than men are. Fortunately, there has been some important research done — especially very recently — on improving women's sexual satisfaction with testosterone therapy. Please notice when we talk about men we speak of "performance", and when we talk about women we speak about "satisfaction". In a search of the entire published literature of the world less than two dozen studies were found for women, while there were hundreds of male studies. Certainly a lot more research is needed on the effects of giving women natural testosterone in small doses for their sexual and other problems and conditions.

We first need to realize that women can have too many or too little androgens in their system. Androgens basically include DHEA, androstenedione and testosterone. Women with too much androgens (androgenicity) suffer from many conditions including facial hair, polycystic ovaries, and various forms of cancer. As always, women need to measure their levels of free testosterone, free androstenedione and DHEA or DHEA-S (sulfate).

A placebo-controlled study at McGill University in Canada (Psychosomatic Medicine 47, 1985, pp. 339-51) looked at women who suffered from surgical menopause after having a hysterectomy (again, the ovaries *always* atrophy and die even if they are not removed). Most all of these women were now testosterone deficient and responded very dramatically to supplementation. "It was clear that exogenous testosterone enhanced the intensity of sexual desire and arousal and frequency of sexual fantasies in hysterectomized and oophorectomized (no ovaries) women." The doctors further said, "The major finding that emerged in this study is that on all three measures of sexual motivation, scores increased concomitant with circulating levels of testosterone." Of course the incompetent doctors injected these unfortunate women with 200 mg of enanthate and should have been imprisoned for such reckless endangerment. They did monitor their blood levels. Coital frequency and orgasmic frequency were not affected however. The truth is that 99 percent of hysterectomies are completely unnecessary in the first place, but that is another matter well discussed in my book, "No More Horse Estrogen!"

Another study at McGill University (Psychoneuro-endocrinology v.18, 1993, pp. 91-102) studied the sexual behavior of younger women and their estradiol, progesterone and free testosterone levels. They found that, "free testosterone was strongly (notice the word 'strongly') and positively associated with sexual desire, sexual thought, and anticipation of sexual activity." They also found testosterone was positively related to attention to sexual stimulation. They concluded, "These results are consistent with the hypothesis that testosterone may enhance cognitive aspects of women's sexual behavior." This is a good and well done study and we need many more like this to understand the effects of hormones in general on the sexual behavior of women.

Further insight on hormones and female sexuality was provided by work at the University of North Carolina (Demography, 23 ,1986, pp. 217-27). Here female adolescents were studied. Levels of testosterone predicted frequency of masturbation (but not frequency of intercourse) for the girls. It was DHEA that did predict how sexually experienced they were. They said, "These (sexual behavior) effects are associated primarily with androgens." And "Hormone effects on female sexual motivation are substantial. These effects are also associated with androgens." However, it was *social* pressure that determined female sexual behavior more than anything.

Another study at the University of North Carolina (Psychosomatic Medicine 59, 1997, pp. 161-71) did the politically incorrect thing of studying the differences between young black and white teenage girls and their sexual behavior. And guess what? They found there are actually racial differences in them! Surprise, surprise! In this study they found that testosterone did predict whether the girls had intercourse earlier in both groups. "Testosterone and changes in testosterone were significantly related to the timing of subsequent transition to first coitus for blacks and whites." They found, "the pubertal rise in testosterone is associated with subsequent increases in female sexual interest and activity." With the white girls again they found social pressure was the controlling factor, and the more the girls attended church the less sex they had and the later they had it. This factor was not significant with the black girls who also had more sexual partners and started at an earlier age. Both groups often denied masturbating which is contrary to known statistics. Testosterone levels actually had predictive value for initiation and frequency of intercourse. Parents may want to saliva test their daughters' levels and keep them locked up if they are on the high side!

Geoffrey Redmond did an interesting review (International Journal of Fertility, v.44, 1999, pp. 193-7). He found that high estrogens can actually decrease libido in women, while androgens are very important for sexual satisfaction. While he prefers overpriced and unnecessary testosterone patches, he doesn't understand that methyl testosterone (!) and injections of salts (50 mg per month!) are Stone Age treatments. Not one time does he state the need for measuring their free levels by blood or saliva analysis and prefers, "monitoring symptoms." He also recommends estradiol supplements generally, although western women generally have *excessive* estrogen levels. As women age they often find a drop in sexual desire and satisfaction in contrast to when they were younger, and doctors who feel like this sure can't help them much.

At the famous Karolinska Institute in Sweden (Climacteric, v. 5, 2002, pp. 357-65) the doctors poisoned women 45-60 years old with oral forty milligram (about 200 times what they needed in their blood) doses of testosterone undecanoate (this is in 2002, remind you) in a double blind study. (Please remember women only produce about 300 micrograms of testosterone a day and need only 150 to 300 mcg of supplemental). All of the women had hysterectomies and/or oophorectomies (removal of the ovaries). One of the most famous clinics in the world isn't competent enough to give women transdermal or sublingual testosterone in normal 150-300 mcg amounts? Nevertheless, they found dramatic effects for sexual relations, especially for satisfaction, frequency and interest in sex. They used the standard McCoy scoring for sexual functioning. They also used the "Psychological General Well Being Index" and found equally dramatic effects for feelings of well being and self esteem. They said, "The addition of testosterone undecanoate improved specific aspects of sexual function." If they had used natural testosterone transdermally or sublingually they would have done much better.

At Utrecht University in the Netherlands (Archives of General Psychiatry, v.57, 2000, pp. 149-53) a unique double blind, placebo study was done on women who were not known to be low in testosterone and were functioning normally. Surprisingly these modern doctors used sublingual testosterone. Only one dose was given to study the effects on physiological and subjective sexual arousal. They gave the women testosterone and then showed them erotic films of couples having intercourse. "The authors found a statistically significant increase in genital responsiveness.

62

Furthermore, on the day of testosterone treatment, there also was a strong and statistically significant association between the increase in genital arousal and subjective reports of genital sensations and sexual lust." Now this is just with one single dose on normal women not known to have any testosterone deficiency at all. This is *not* to infer that any woman with normal levels should in any way consider raising them to supraphysiological (i.e. excessive) levels. High levels of androgens cause serious conditions in women just as deficient levels do.

A very surprising study was done almost thirty years ago at three hospitals in the United Kingdom (British Journal of Psychiatry, v. 132, 1978, pp. 339-46). Sexually unresponsive women were studied along with their husbands and given counseling since sexuality is more psychological than physiological. Amazingly enough they were given sublingual testosterone! The fact that women were given the proper sublingual form almost three decades ago is a credit to these researchers. Unfortunately, however, they were given huge, toxic 10 mg doses (about thirty times too much), but only for ninety days. One third of one milligram would be good. The results were nothing less than dramatic, including frequency of orgasm, arousal, erotic feelings, and satisfaction. "Those receiving testosterone did significantly better on a number of behavioral and attitudinal measures…." Not only was their sexual happiness greatly improved, but their overall psychology as well.

A dozen doctors from around the country collaborated (New England Journal of Medicine, v. 343, 2000, pp. 682-8) to study women after removal of their ovaries. There is very little testosterone produced by the adrenal glands after a hysterectomy or oophorectomy. Sexual functioning in these women is severely impaired. One third of all American women will suffer unnecessary hysterectomy at an average age of only forty years. The women were given 150-300 mcg of transdermal testosterone daily since their rate of production is only about 600 mcg a day. "In women who had undergone oophorectomy, transdermal testosterone improves sexual function and psychological well being." The doctors went on to say, "…as reflected by scores on the "Brief   Index of Sexual Functioning for Women," the dimensions of thoughts (desire, arousal, frequency of sexual activity, pleasure and orgasm) were most affected." While sexual satisfaction was dramatically improved, their general psychology was equally affected. "In regard to psychological status, testosterone replacement had a beneficial effect on well-being and depressed mood." When natural testosterone is given in natural ways the effects are no less than stunning.

NIMH (National Institutes of Mental Health) sponsored a study almost three decades ago (Archives of Sexual Behavior, v. 7, 1978, pp. 157-73) showing the relationship of testosterone levels in women to sexual satisfaction. Young, healthy married couples were extensively studied with in-depth psychological tests as well as hormone measurements. "The wives' self-rated gratification scores correlated significantly with their own plasma testosterone levels….that high baseline testosterone level was significantly related to high self-rated gratification score and to ability to form good interpersonal relationships." Not only was sexual satisfaction related to testosterone levels but the very ability to have a better relationship with other people. It was also pointed out that low testosterone was related to anxiety and high testosterone to freedom from anxiety.

There's not much more the worldwide published literature over the last three decades has to offer us on the influence of testosterone for female sexuality. This is changing and most of these studies were done in the last five years. Ladies, you don't need any more studies. Just test your free testosterone and supplement it if you are low. If you are too high just change your diet and lifestyle to lower your level. Please read my books *No More Horse Estrogen!* and *Zen Macrobiotics for Americans.*

Chapter 12: Male Sexuality

The published literature on male sexuality is overwhelming and mostly concerns erectile dysfunction. Again, we always see "performance" in men, and "satisfaction" in women. Science proves that testosterone and androgens in general are very important to sexual function in men, but far down the list as to causing impotence. Testosterone supplementation is only going to help sexually dysfunctional men who are very low in this hormone. We'll concentrate on measurement of testosterone and use of transdermal forms rather than the usual injections or oral use of synthetic salts.

A very good study came from the famous Karolinska Institute in 1996 (Journal of Urology, v. 155, pp. 1604-8). Hypogonadal men aged 21-65 were given transdermal patches that delivered 5 mg a day of natural testosterone (only about 20% penetration rate and very expensive). These doctors are to be given a lot of credit for using natural testosterone transdermally in normal doses. These patches raised their free testosterone levels to youthful levels without raising estrogens or DHT. They gave these men extensive subjective and objective tests of various kinds to monitor their improvement. They concluded, "...nocturnal erections occurred more frequently with longer duration and greater rigidity, and patient assessments of sexual desire and weekly number of erections were higher." They said further, "These findings suggest that androgen replacement therapy has an impact on all aspects of male sexual function, unconscious and conscious." They quoted a number of other studies that found similar results. Research like this will eventually result in testosterone testing and supplementation in normal routine medical practice instead of symptomatic and unnatural chemical band-aids like Viagra®, Levitra®, and Cialis®. Remember though, this was a great improvement and not a cure-all by any means.

At the Association pour l'"Etude de la Pathologie in France (Journal of Urology, v. 158, 1997, pp. 1964-7) we find out just how little the medical profession knows about hormones. 1,022 men complaining of erectile dysfunction (ED) were studied and their testosterone measured. The doctors arbitrarily decided that any man with a level of less than 4 ng/ml was testosterone deficient. This meant that only 9 percent (one in eleven) men over the age of fifty were deemed hypogonadal and in need of supplementation. Folks, the facts of the matter are that at least 90 percent of men over the age of fifty are testosterone deficient and could benefit greatly from supplementation. Calling the worst 9 percnet the cutoff point is ridiculous. To use a sickly, but technically average, standard like this makes no sense at all. Low levels found in aging men may be "normal" for their age, but are nevertheless pathological and cause serious problems. The *youthful* levels men enjoyed at about the age of thirty should always be the standard. They used both testosterone heptylate (a toxic and unnatural injected salt) and human chorionic gonadotropin (HCG) to raise testosterone levels!!!!! Again, even using the wrong type in the wrong ways resulted in impressive benefits. They did find good success with erectile dysfunction but only with the men with the lowest testosterone levels. Again, we see that sex is 90 percent psychology and only 10 percent biology in men.

At the University of Modena in Italy (International Journal of Andrology, v. 19, 1996, pp. 48-54 and Journal of Andrology, v. 18, 1997 pp. 522-7) two studies were done. In the first, healthy men were divided into four groups according to their testosterone level. Only the lowest group showed problems as reflected by nocturnal electronic monitoring of their erections. "Group 1 showed significantly impaired night erections when compared with any of the other three groups, but no differences were detected among groups 2, 3 and 4." In the second, healthy subjects were divided into eight groups according to their testosterone level. Their erections during sleep were also monitored electronically. "The groups of subjects with higher testosterone serum levels (400 ng and above) showed almost constantly higher value for the erectile parameters studied than the subjects with serum testosterone less than

99 ng/dL." It must be pointed out that only the men with the lowest testosterone levels had serious problems with nocturnal erections so the majority of men will not be helped by such therapy.

At the well-known Kinsey Institute of Research (Psycho-neuroendocrinology, v. 20, 1995, pp. 743-53) a double blind study with normal and hypogonadal men was done. They were given erotic stimuli and their erections monitored electronically. "The number of satisfactory nocturnal penile tumescence (nighttime erections) responses, in terms of both circumfrence increase and rigidity, were less in the hypogonadal men than the controls and were significantly increased by androgen replacement, confirming the results of earlier studies." There was good improvement here, but only in the hypogonadal men. Testosterone is only one factor, albeit a major factor is male sexual performance and ability.

Some important, extensive, and comprehensive work was done at Boston University in 1994 (Journal of Urology, v. 151, pp. 54-61). This was the famous Massachusetts Male Aging Study (MMAS) on 1,290 average men aged 40-70. Fully 10 percent of these men were impotent and 52 percent suffered from transient or partial impotence. *One in ten men over the age of forty in America cannot function sexually*! Over half of them have serious problems with sexual performance. The older the men were the more promi-nent their sexual dysfunction. They found the causative factors to be *age*, heart disease, hypertension, diabetes, prescription medica-tion, anger, depression, high cholesterol, cigarette smoking, and low DHEA levels. Seventeen hormones were measured in these men and only low DHEA was related to impotence. Testosterone, including free testosterone, was not found to be a factor at all sur-prisingly. There are no simple or easy cures for male sexual dys-function. Alcoholics functioned just fine for some reason, as did obese and arthritic men. This epidemic of impotence is largely hidden because of the shame these men feel about their condition. This is due to *lifestyle* obviously more than anything else.

Impressed by the above study, doctors at the University of Vienna looked at men with erectile dysfunction (ED) for their hormone levels (Urology, v. 53, 1999, pp. 590-5). They also found that low DHEA was a major cause of impotence. "Our results suggest that oral DHEA treatment may be of benefit in the treatment of ED." It becomes obvious that both testosterone and DHEA should be measured and supplemented if necessary in men over 40 or younger men with sexual functioning problems. (Androstenedione generally tracks testosterone and very rarely needs to be supplemented by itself).

Doctors at Northwestern University did a fine review and meta-analysis of 16 major studies chosen from 73 published ones (Journal of Urology, v. 164, 2000, pp. 371-5). "Our meta-analysis of the usefulness of androgen replacement therapy for erectile dysfunction indicates that the response rate for a primary etiology was improved over that for a secondary etiology, transdermal testosterone therapy was more effective than intramuscular or oral treatment..." They found 81 percent of men treated with transdermal forms got benefits, but this sounds very optimistic. They pointed out that erectile dysfunction, while too embarrassing to be openly discussed, affects up to thrity million American men.

Impotence and sexual dysfunction in men is a hidden problem they are not willing to admit to or discuss openly. Synthetic chemicals such as Viagra®, Cialis®, and Levitra® are not the answer at all, don't work in most men, and merely deal with the superficial symptom of much deeper problems. We will not discuss the many dozens of studies around the world over the last twenty years that used injections or oral doses of toxic salts. Yes, the patients nearly always got impressive benefits, but only if they were very low in free testosterone. Fortunately doctors are slowly waking up to the fact that the correct way to administer non-oral hormones like testosterone (progesterone, estriol and growth hormone) is transdermally or sublingually. Sexuality is a complex situation and hormones are only one part of this especially in men. It is your total *lifestyle* that causes — and cures — impotence, not "magic hormones."

Chapter 13: Women Need Testosterone, Too

It is well known that women are more influenced by their hormones than men are. This is certainly true when it comes to testosterone. Although women only have about one tenth the amount of blood testosterone men do, it is no less important to them. It is estimated that women produce about 300 mcg a day but retain more of it in their blood than men do. Just because they have a lower level of blood testosterone does not mean it has any less effect on them. Medical doctors have no idea how important testosterone is for women and almost never test them for their levels, much less prescribe supplements for them. The traditional wisdom is that testosterone is, "the male hormone" and estrogen the female hormone. Even if doctors did measure female androgens, they would have no idea of the difference between their bound, total, and free levels, and even less idea of how to properly administer it to those who are deficient. In the entire scientific world there are only a handful of published studies (most very recently) on testosterone therapy for women, few of which use natural testosterone transdermally or sublingually.

Ladies, if you have some idea you are going to visit your local physician who will help you with this, you are very, very mistaken. You may have to find a holistically oriented physician who will even be willing to write you a testosterone prescription. Normal pharmacies can't help you. One way to do this is to ask the local compounding pharmacist which doctors are writing prescriptions for transdermal or sublingual testosterone for men and women. First, test your saliva level to see if you are low and if you require supplementation. The doctor will still insist on a blood test, so demand that he only test your free, bioavailable level; do not pay for unnecessary total and bound testing. We like to think we are technologically advanced, especially in America, but when it comes to health we are often in the Dark Ages. Yes, there are Estratest® patches available for women with estrogen and toxic methyl testosterone. This is the same methyl testosterone recom-

69

mended in one insane book for women on testosterone "therapy". *Never* take toxic, unnatural methyl testosterone due to the severe side effects! There are patches available for women that deliver 150 mcg of natural testosterone daily but, again, these are inordinately expensive, especially for women, since there is so little actual hormone in these. You may pay $100 a month for literally twenty-five cents worth of testosterone. Buy your own testosterone on the Internet from foreign online pharmacies. Let's look at some of the very, very few studies that do exist.

At Massachusetts General Hospital collaborating with other clinics (New England Journal of Medicine, v. 343, 2000, pp. 682-8) researchers gave transdermal testosterone to women who had their ovaries removed (oophorectomy). The ovaries supply about half the testosterone in women while the adrenal glands supply the other half. Some of the women got 150 mcg and others got 300 mcg of natural testosterone from expensive transdermal patches. Applying one-gram daily of a 0.3 percent cream or gel is just as effective at a fraction of the price. The loss of uterine and ovarian function has severe physical and mental side effects that are played down by the medical profession. Most doctors actually consider the uterus a useless organ with no function after childbirth or menopause! The women were given extensive psychological and physical testing. The women's psychological well being, depression, and sexual function improved dramatically with either dose. Frequency of sexual activity, coital dysfunction, pleasure and enjoyment, as well as orgasm were much improved. "In women who had undergone oophorectomy and hysterectomy transdermal testosterone improves sexual function and psychological well-being." It seems the 150mcg dose was more beneficial than the higher 300 mcg (two patch) dose. We should always remember that excessive androgens in women are deleterious. Doctors like this deserve a lot of credit for their ground-breaking work and this is first rate work.

At the Jean Hailes Foundation in Australia (Trends in Endocrinology and Metabolism, v. 12, 2001, pp. 33-7) we find somewhat less enlightened research. Here the female doctors recommend injections of nandrolone, which is an unnatural synthetic

70

analog of testosterone with serious side effects. This kind of ignorance and irresponsibility is simply inexcusable since natural testosterone is inexpensive and widely available. Other methods of supplementation including real transdermal testosterone were discussed. The fact that women would do this to other women is appalling.

At Baylor College the doctors were even worse. They said that oral methyl testosterone, "is the most commonly used form of androgen replacement for postmenopausal women." (International Journal of Fertility, v. 41, 1996, pp. 412-22). Methyl testosterone is the worst possible form of testosterone and is extremely toxic and dangerous. This should be completely banned for human or animal use. Any doctor who gives a person methyl testosterone should be imprisoned, sued, and their medical license permanently revoked. These doctors also try to convince us that testosterone in women actually rises with age. The facts are (as you can see by the charts on page 20 of this book) that testosterone falls until menopause and then rises slightly, but stays far below youthful levels. This is obviously the kind of "research" we don't need.

To show more doctors who are out of touch with current research we only need to look at a study from Vienna Medical University in Austria (Obstetrics and Gynecology, v. 89, 1997, pp. 297-9). These poor women were given transdermal testosterone, but 1) they used the synthetic, unnatural propionate ester rather than real natural testosterone, and 2) they gave the women 40 mg a day!!!! If only 10 percent of this was absorbed (it was in petroleum which is a very ineffective base for skin penetration) this would mean 4,000 mcg instead of a reasonable 150 mcg. This is a one-month supply every day or almost *thirty* times what they needed. Almost all of the women were immediately well over the high range and started to develop serious side effects. To make things worse they did not limit the supplementary testosterone to women who had low levels, but gave it to all the women in the study regardless of their level.

One of the very few good reviews on women and testosterone was done at the University of Utah in 2002 with an impressive 56 references (International Journal of Fertility, v. 47, pp. 77-86). It was pointed out that women only produce about 300 mcg a day (one third of one milligram), half of this from the ovaries and half from the adrenals. Contrary to logic, a few women after hysterectomy still have excessive testosterone levels even though their ovaries have atrophied (regardless of whether or not they were removed). They discuss "Female Androgen Deficiency Syndrome" or FADS. The researchers here show that testosterone falls strongly between the ages of 20-50 prior to menopause, but rises somewhat after menopause.

One third of American women will needlessly suffer from a hysterectomy at an average age of only forty years. This senseless procedure is somehow accepted as normal. If doctors tried to castrate one third of the men in this country they would all be hung the next day. Why do women so passively agree to be castrated for no valid reason? Ladies, please read such books as *No More Hysterectomies*, *The Hysterectomy Hoax*, and *The Castrated Woman*. At UCLA in San Diego (American Journal of Obstetrics and Gynecology, v. 118, 1974, pp. 793-8) thirty years ago women with endometrial cancer had their ovaries removed. Their testosterone and androstenedione levels fell to less than half immediately after the operation. Their DHEA also fell but was not measured. No attempt was made to supplement their deficient levels nor was the concept even addressed! To add insult to injury they were then injected with synthetic toxic medroxyprogesterone instead of being given natural transdermal progesterone. Why aren't women with deficient hormone levels after hysterectomy routinely given supplemental natural hormones?

Most all American women suffer from PMS and some rather severely. At NIH in Maryland in 1998 (Biological Psychiatry, v. 43, pp. 897-903) women with PMS and low testosterone levels were compared to healthy controls. PMS is the most common female complaint and the symptoms can last for up to fifteen years after the menses cease. "PMS subjects had significantly lower total and free plasma testosterone levels with a blunting of the normal periovulatory peak, a finding that may be epiphenomenal (related) to age." This is not to suggest that supplemental testosterone is a "magic cure" for PMS, nor even that all women with PMS are testosterone deficient, but rather it is an important factor that needs to be addressed. PMS is epidemic in Western cultures, but not in Asian or African cultures. Women suffering from PMS can cure this by changing their diets and balancing their progesterone, estriol, DHEA, T3, T4, and pregnenolone in addition to their testosterone.

Another study from Hope Hospital in England in 1998 (Clinical Endocrinology, v. 49, pp. 173-8) came to the same conclusions. Women with severe PMS (average age of 40) were given under the skin (s.c.) silastic implants of natural testosterone. These implants slowly release 100 mg of the hormone every six months for over two years. This is expensive and very unnecessary, but does, in fact, use natural testosterone delivered in reasonable amounts. Plasma levels rose from an average of 237 percent, which is definitely excessive. They found this regimen to be safe and without side effects with good improvement in the short term. Imagine the improvement if they had addressed all their basic hormones. The silastic implants are not practical means to do this since they need surgical implantation, are unnecessary, and very expensive. The doctors were concerned about the long-term safety of low-dose androgen supplementation for women, but found, "Overall, this study provides largely reassuring data about the safety of low-dose androgen treatment in women. No patient experienced adverse symptoms while on testosterone treatment."

More and more doctors are realizing that androgens such as DHEA, testosterone and androstenedione are vital to the health and well being of women and are not merely "male hormones". Australian researchers (Clinical Endocrinology & Metabolism, v. 17, 2003, pp. 165-75) did a review with many references on testosterone therapy for women. "Clinical symptoms of androgen insufficiency (in women) include loss of libido, diminished well-being, fatigue and blunted motivation and have been reported to respond well to testosterone replacement, generally without significant side effects." It is doctors like this that will help women maintain their natural hormone balance throughout life, instead of poisoning them with horse estrogen and synthetic progestins.

Finally in 2004 the medical profession provided some much needed light on the subject of androgens for female health. The entire supplement of Mayo Clinic Proceedings (v. 79) was devoted to this subject. We will cover all five studies:

At Columbia University "Formulations and Use of Androgens in Women" was submitted. They reported that the most common symptoms of female testosterone deficiency are decreased libido and sexual pleasure, low energy and fatigue, anxiety, lack of motivation, diminished sense of well being, decreased bone density, diminished muscle mass, increase in body fat, less cognitive ability and memory loss. They recognized the need for routine measurement of free testosterone in women and supplementation when necessary. Unfortunately they feel methyl testosterone is a valid means of administration as well as the overpriced patches, oral salts, and injected salts. They do see promise in sublingual, vaginal, and transdermal gels to their credit.

At Adult Women's Health and Medicine in Florida an article on hot flashes was submitted. Hot flashes are all too common for premenopausal and menopausal women especially in European countries. (This is not true in Asian and African countries generally.) Testosterone therapy is suggested for this very popular problem. Again, methyl testosterone is recommended as a valid means of administration, which shows good intentions are not always matched by intelligence, competence nor capability.

At the Mayo Clinic itself bone health was studied in relation to female testosterone levels. This has already been covered in the Osteoporosis and Bone Health chapter. Osteoporosis is epidemic in European women, but not so much in Asian, African or Latin women in their indigenous countries. Instead of treating bone mineral density deficiency with toxic, ineffective, expensive and symptomatic prescription drugs we should be doing this with natural hormones like testosterone and progesterone and supplements like glucosamine, minerals, and vitamin D.

The fourth study from Harvard Medical School was "The Role of Androgens in Female Sexual Dysfunction". This has already been covered in the Female Sexuality chapter. "The role of low androgen concentration in female sexual dysfunction is gaining increasing attention....and early clinical trial results suggest that they may be both effective and safe in the treatment of FSD, specifically low libido." They point out that a survey of thousands of American women aged 18 to 59 (Journal of the American Medical Association, v. 281, 1999, pp. 1174) that a full 43 percent reported serious sexual dysfunction — almost half!

The last study was on safety and side effects from Johns Hopkins University. Unfortunately it was oriented around "risks" and "side effects" instead of benefits. They pointed out that using methyl testosterone (the most commonly prescribed form for American women), nandrolone (a dangerous analog), and injectable salts have side effects. It was admitted that transdermal gel, natural implant pellets and patches do not have these problems. If doctors would just realize that natural testosterone used in natural ways in women proven to be deficient literally has *no side effects whatsoever* and is completely safe, they would finally understand the situation. When transdermal or sublingual testosterone is used in the proper amounts there are never any side effects. Women suffering from hyperandrogenism were also discussed. Excessive testosterone levels in women can only be lowered by diet, exercise, supplements and lifestyle — not by toxic prescription drugs.

Some good work was done at the Kinsey Institute (Clinical Endocrinology, v. 45, 1996, pp. 577-87) on androgens in women after menopause. Women will live the last third of their lives after their menses cease. The menopausal transition is problematic for the vast majority of Western women. These problems (such as osteoporosis, memory loss, body fat, etc.) persist throughout the rest of their lives. Women 40-60 years of age were studied to see the endocrine changes after menopause for estradiol, estrone, progesterone, LH, FSH, testosterone, androstenedione, DHEA, cortisol and even BMI. There were no easy answers or pat generalizations here. Each woman had a distinct and unique endocrine profile that must be addressed individually by testing each of her hormones.

Because one in three American women suffer from a hysterectomy and their entire hormone balance upset, we need to review the few studies done on them. At McGill University in Canada (American Journal of Obstetrics and Gynecology, v. 151, 1985, pp. 153-60) women were given supplemental testosterone after hysterectomy. They were evaluated with an index of twenty-six common symptoms. "The superior efficacy of the androgen-containing preparations on somatic, psychological and total scores of the menopausal index may also be relation to the anabolic and energizing properties of this sex steroid (testosterone)."

Women reading this book should also read my *No More Horse Estrogen!* to learn more about natural health for women. Surgery and drugs are obviously not the answer for female health problems. Diet, proven supplements, natural hormone balance, avoidance of bad habits, exercise, and even fasting and meditation are the answer. Natural health is about diet and lifestyle more than anything else. The more women take responsibility for their own health and stay away from doctors the better off they will be. As more women look at the very causes of their health problems and not try to cover up the outward symptoms they will be able to prevent and cure their illnesses. The medical profession is going to be decades catching the fact that women need youthful levels of androstenedione, DHEA and testosterone. Any woman can basically test and balance her own hormone levels with inexpensive saliva kits without a doctor. There are almost no medical doctors or gynecologists in the world who have any ability at all to help with natural hormone testing and supplementation. Take responsibility for your own health and wellbeing, ladies.

Chapter 14: Psychology and Behavior

One of the countless insanities in our culture is to give people toxic, unnatural, dangerous mind numbing drugs if they are depressed, anxious, or have other psychological problems. God forbid that we treat the whole person and their lifestyle to understand what is causing their unhappiness and deal with that. Our basic hormones have a very strong influence on our moods, outlook, and feelings of well being, especially in women. Unfortunately, most of the studies on testosterone's influence on mood and behavior have been done on men. In the future we will see much more work on how hormones influence psychology on women.

A fine study was done at the University of Connecticut in 2002 (Journals of Gerontology, v. 57A, pp. M321-5). Here real natural transdermal testosterone was given to hypogonadal depressed men. Only 5 mg of testosterone per day was delivered via patches (a cream or gel would have been more practical and less expensive). Their free testosterone levels went from a mere 93-163 on the average, while estrone and estradiol were basically unchanged. That is how thorough they were. They also cited thirty-five references that demonstrated how male psychology can be impaired by low testosterone levels. They said, "Testosterone levels in older men may positively influence health perception associated with perceived physical function." This is science as it should be.

A very interesting study was done at UCLA in Torrance in 1996 (Journal of Clinical Endocrinology & Metabolism, v. 81, p. 3578-83). Here men aged 22-60 with low testosterone were either given injections of testosterone enanthate (TE), a unique 7.5 mg sublingual natural testosterone (SLT) solution, or 15 mg of SLT. All the men generally reduced their feelings of anger, sadness, irritability, tiredness and nervousness. They increased their feelings of friendliness, good feelings and energy. The men given the TE injections were very overdosed and their testosterone level fluctuated severely between injections every 20 days. Nevertheless they also got dramatic results. The men given the 15 mg of SLT were also very overdosed. The men given the unique 7.5 mg (3 to 5 mg would have been safer) SLT basically normalized their testosterone. Something very suspicious here is that the estradiol (E2) levels were measured before and after the administration and they refused to reveal these levels! Obviously this is because the TE injections caused severe rises in E2 and the 15 mg SLT caused large rises. To refuse to reveal the known E2 levels is inexcusable. The lesson to be learned from this study is that low dose SLT therapy is an excellent way to deliver testosterone in both men and women. How supposed professionals can be so smart, yet overlook the obvious at the same time, is hard to comprehend.

At Drew University in Los Angeles in 1996 (Journal of Clinical Endocrinology & Metabolism, v. 81, pp. 3754-8) some completely irresponsible doctors gave men aged 19 to 40 with *normal* testosterone levels a ridiculous 600 mg of injected testosterone enanthate (TE) every week to force their levels far beyond normal. Of course their estrone and estradiol levels went through the roof, but they refused to address that vital situation - they didn't even bother to measure them! They did this to find out whether very high, out of range testosterone levels cause anger and aggression. They found out it definitely did not and this is a very important finding. Stories of bodybuilders who experienced "'roid rage" are due to artificial, dangerous steroids and not testosterone. Doctors like this should have their licenses revoked and imprisoned after being sued for gross negligence.

A valuable study in 2003 from Harvard Medical School (American Journal of Psychiatry, v. 160, pp. 105-11) used natural transdermal gel in men aged 30 to 65 who suffered from depression. The problem here was they gave them a preposterous 10 g of a 1% gel which equates to 100 mg of actual testosterone applied to the skin! Remember that hypogonadal men only need about 3-4 mg a day actually delivered into their system as they only produce about 6-8 mg a day. Another problem was that they did not even bother to measure their estrone or estradiol levels, which obviously went off the scale from such overdosing. One would think Harvard doctors had some common sense or basic knowledge of hormone metabolism. Anyway, the men responded splendidly and largely overcame their feelings of depression. Even when given too much testosterone the benefits were very dramatic and proven by multiple psychological testing such as the Beck Depression Inventory, Hamilton Depression Rating Scale and Clinical Global Impression.

A very impressive and extensive review was done at the Munster University in Germany with a long list of 222 references in 2001 (European Journal of Endocrinology, v. 144, p.183-97). Stress lowers testosterone and stress is epidemic in Western society. Dealing with stress successfully allows the natural testosterone level to rise. Aggressive behavior was not attributed to high testosterone levels. Synthetic anabolic weightlifter steroids have been shown to cause anger and aggressiveness, however. Even giving men excessive doses of supplemental testosterone did not increase their anger or aggression levels. It is depression in men that has clearly been linked to low testosterone levels. We need to study women to see if this has any bearing on them. Depressed hypogonadal men should be treated with supplemental testosterone rather than given mind numbing, dangerous, toxic psychoactive drugs with severe side effects.

A study from the University of Western Ontario in 1996 (Aggressive Behavior, v. 22, pp. 321-31) showed different results, however. Both male and female young students had their free, salivary testosterone measured. "Within each sex, testosterone was positively correlated with aggression and negatively correlated with pro-social personality." Men somehow only had five times the blood testosterone level of women instead of the usual ten to one ratio. We all know men and women have different cognitive abilities. Men are better with math and women are better with verbal skills. Musical skills are negatively correlated with testosterone in men but positively correlated in women. We need to study social status and testosterone in both men and women as there are indications this has significant relevance. Yes, there are racial differences contrary to liberal political correctness. Asians generally have the highest testosterone levels, Africans moderate levels with

Europeans the lowest levels. Other aspects of this well done review will be discussed in the appropriate chapters.

While going through *every* single published study on women and testosterone in the last twenty years in Chemical Abstracts it was almost impossible to find any such research in the entire world. There are just very few published studies anywhere in the world as testosterone is still considered, "the male hormone". It is hard to understand why medical doctors cannot see how important testosterone is for women. We need to do such research especially since women are more hormonally driven than men are.

A review done at Essen University in Germany in 2002 (Maturitas, v. 41, pp. S25-46) showed the same basic relationship with depression and low testosterone in women. This twenty-two page review had a full 137 cited references. Doctor Uwe Rohr is an excellent example of what progressive researchers should be doing. This also showed that excessive testosterone is related to depression (men cannot naturally have excessive levels). Women suffer from depression more than men do, so this is much more important to them. Testosterone levels fall about 50 percent generally in women by menopause (some women, on the other hand, suffer from androgenicity and excessive levels.) Hypoandrogenism in women is related to depression, osteoporosis, low libido, genital atrophy and higher body fat levels. Hyperandrogenism in women is related to hirstutism (body and facial hair), acne and polycystic ovaries - which is epidemic in American women. This study further divided the women into four groups of testosterone to estradiol ratios for such risk categories as diabetes, cancer and CHD disease. There is a wealth of information in this review that is far too comprehensive to go into in detail.

At the University of Utah two studies were published including a review in 1995 complete with forty-three references (Hormones and Behavior, v. 29, pp. 354-66 and Aggressive Behavior, v. 29, 2003, pp. 107-115) on status, self-regard, competitiveness, aggression, assertiveness and dominance in young women in relation to testosterone levels. DHEA and estradiol were not found to have any relationships to behavior. They did, however, find a definite correlation between these factors as they relate to testosterone levels. Women with higher testosterone levels who ranked themselves well in status were not considered to have higher status by their peers though. One other study also showed confident, uninhibited and action-oriented behavior to be correlated with higher testosterone levels in young women. Still another study found just the opposite, however, while others have shown no relationship at all. There are no easy answers here. Occupational status and testosterone in women have shown the same inconsistencies. This is complicated by the fact that some occupations require assertiveness while others require other traits. A woman lawyer or saleswoman might benefit from such behavior, while a nurse or teacher would not. Societal norms would also be important here. An Asian or Muslim woman might fare poorly with aggressive and assertive behavior, while an American woman could fare very well in many areas. Testosterone was positively associated with self-regard (ranking themselves in their peer group), and dominant behavior - as well as their number of sexual partners. It was inversely associated with smiling, so there is an obvious price to pay for such self-assuredness.

The Rancho Bernardo Study in 1999 (Journal of Clinical Endocrinology & Metabolism, v. 84, pp. 573-7) was some of the most important research ever done but was only concerned with men unfortunately. Over eight hundred hypogonadal men over the age of 50 had their bioavailable testosterone measured. They were then administered the Beck Depression Inventory. There was no doubt about the strong relationship between their hormone levels and states of depression. "These results suggest that testosterone treatment might improve depressed mood in older men who have low levels of bioavailable testosterone." These very same doctors should now study older women for the same phenomenon and include other hormones such as estrone and estradiol.

One might think that sensation seekers of both sexes would have higher testosterone levels, but this doesn't seem to be true. A study at Florida State University in 2001 (Hormones and Behavior,

81

v. 40, pp. 396-402) tested young college men and women for their testosterone and cortisol levels. No relationship at all was found for testosterone and sensation seeking behavior such as sky diving, bungee jumping, water skiing, roller coaster riding and the like. However, low cortisol in men (but not in women) was found to be linked to risky behavior or the desire for such behavior.

At the National Institute of Aging in 2002 (Journal of Clinical Endocrinology & Metabolism, v. 87, pp. 5001-7) men were given sophisticated psychological tests. It was clear that older men over 50 with higher testosterone fared much better than their hypogonadal counterparts in regard to memory, stress, cognitive function, depression and other related factors.

At the German Central Institute of Mental Health in 2000 (Psychoneuroendocrinology, v. 25, pp. 765-71) women aged 28 to 77 were studied for depression as it related to their androgen levels. They noticed, "To date, there is only sparse information about the regulation of androstenedione, testosterone and DHT (dihydro-testosterone) concentrations in women with severe major depression." What an understatement! Here they found estradiol unrelated, but excessive levels of testosterone, androstenedione and DHT clearly related to depression. They also found generally low testosterone in the depressed women as well as hyper levels.

At the University of Lubeck in Germany (Neuro-psychopharmacology, v. 28, 2003, pp.1538-45) women aged 47 to 65 were given supplemental testosterone to show the effects on their "divergent and covergent" thought processes. They found that testosterone strongly affects the thought process in women especially pre-menopausal women who have higher levels during ovulation. Here we demonstrate empirically how women are very hormonally influenced physically, mentally and emotionally and why we need more knowledge about endocrine effects on their thoughts and feelings.

Chapter 15: Obesity and BMI

America is the most overweight country in the world. We not only eat more calories than anyone else, but more empty, nutritionless calories, 160 pounds of various sugars annually, and 42 percent of our caloric intake as fat — especially saturated animal fats. Overfed and undernourished. We also get less exercise than anyone else on earth. We don't need to wonder why we're so overweight. There are no shortcuts or "magic answers" to weight loss. Will power is an illusion, as you can't deny hunger instinct. Diet and lifestyle is the key to staying slim all your life. You can literally eat all you want if you eat whole, healthy natural foods. Please read my book, *Zen Macrobiotics for Americans*.

Yes, hormones do play an important part in this in addition to diet and exercise. Androgen deficiency as well as low thyroid (T3 and T4) and high estrogens (estradiol and estrone) are especially important to metabolic rate. As you would expect, there was quite a lot of research done on obesity regarding men, but almost none on women. As always, women should have a normal, youthful range of androgens avoiding both hyper- and hypo- levels. Youthful testosterone levels are vital to maintaining slimness and a low body mass index (BMI), but this is only one part of a total program of diet, exercise and lifestyle. Expect some changes in your BMI and body fat percent from maintaining a youthful testosterone (and DHEA) level, but not any dramatic ones. Your best results will come from realizing all your hormones work together as a team. You must balance your other basic hormones to get the most effect. Definitely you should test your free T3 and free T4 (not your TSH or T3 uptake) thyroid hormones since these affect your metabolic rate so strongly. Do *not* accept low normal levels here, but keep them at least at mid-range. DHEA is your other major androgen and also important in maintaining slimness. Keep a youthful level of DHEA. Men can test for excessive estradiol and estrone and women can test for these as well as for estriol (estriol is rarely out of balance in men). Be sure to balance your pregnenolone and melatonin as well. Growth hormone is important, but simply too expensive at $1,200 a year minimum (for Chinese Jintropin®). You can expect to gain some lean muscle mass, but controlling percentage of body fat is a more difficult matter. Some studies find loss of body fat, while others find no changes when supplemental testosterone is given.

A very informative study was done at the University of Munster in 2002 (European Journal of Endocrinology, v. 146, pp. 505-11) which was previously discussed in Chapter 4. Here they used oral, injected, and transdermal (patches) forms on hypogonadal men. There was very insightful information here about BMI and testosterone levels as men age. They concluded that, "...testosterone appears to be an important factor contributing to these changes. Thus aging men should benefit from testosterone substitution as far as body composition is concerned." The fall in testosterone as men age was paralleled by a rise in BMI and body fat mass. This was reduced significantly by raising testosterone levels, even when using the wrong types in the wrong ways. Leptin was also found to increase with age and BMI, but this could be due to leptin resistance. With all the research on leptin there still has not been any practical means found to raise or lower it to change the composition of the body. Normal men gained BMI, body fat, and leptin as they aged, but lost testosterone. Men given supplemental testosterone did not gain BMI, body fat, or leptin and kept youthful testosterone levels. The authors, unfortunately, somehow felt only "20-30 percent" of aging men had subnormal testosterone levels, when the well proven facts show over 90 percent of them do. All this should equally apply to women basically.

Rising leptin levels as related to age were studied at the University of Koln in Germany in 1997 (Journal of Clinical Endocrinology & Metabolism, v. 82, p. 2510-3) correlating it with falling testosterone and rising BMI. Low leptin levels correlated with slimness, and high leptin levels correlated with obesity. (Men have lower leptin levels than women.) The hypogonadal men in this study had three times the leptin levels of the normal subjects. Therefore an inverse relationship exists where low testosterone and high leptin help cause obesity. There is every reason to think the same situation would occur in women. "We conclude that hypogonadal men exhibit elevated leptin levels that are normalized by substitution with testosterone."

At the National School of Public Health in Athens (Annals of Nutrition and Metabolism, v. 43, 1999, pp. 23-9) healthy elderly men were studied for their body mass and their hormone levels. Not surprisingly they found that low testosterone was equated with obesity and high testosterone equated with slimness. They also found higher estradiol levels equated with obesity and low estradiol with slimness. They also studied leptin. High leptin was associated with obesity and low leptin with slimness. Of course they found the higher the leptin levels the lower the testosterone levels. They also found the more dietary fat the men ate the higher their leptin levels — and the lower their testosterone.

At the University of Pennsylvania School of Medicine (Journal of Clinical Endocrinology and Metabolism, v. 84, 1999, pp. 2647-53) elderly men were given real transdermal testosterone. Of course all of these men were low in testosterone since they were all over the age of sixty-five. This was a true double blind study where half the men were given placebo patches. This study lasted a full three years. The men lost an average of almost seven pounds of ugly fat while making no changes at all in their diet or lifestyle. They gained almost five pounds of real muscle. When you lose fat and gain muscle your total body mass is exponentially improved. This was all done by simply raising their testosterone naturally to youthful levels and not asking them to do anything else at all. Imagine what they could have done with more hormone balance, a better diet and some reasonable exercise!

At the University of Vermont (Journal of Clinical Endocrinology and Metabolism, v. 81, 1996, pp. 3469-75) hypogonadal men aged 33 to 57 were given injections of 300 mg of testosterone cyprionate every two weeks. Even though they were given the wrong kind of testosterone in the wrong way they still got dramatic effects. Just think of how much better they would have fared if given natural testosterone in a natural way. Their free testosterone level went up strongly, but only temporarily, and fell back down to deficient levels before the next injection. The good doctors refused to measure estradiol and estrone levels, which went up just as strongly after the injections. Their actual gain of real muscle was an amazing 15 percent. The loss of ugly fat was a stunning 11 percent. When you add the muscle gain to the fat loss this is really impressive especially since they made no dietary or exercise changes. The men actually gained a small amount of weight in that they were now more muscular. "We conclude that testosterone replacement in hypogonadal men enhanced the skeletal muscle mass by stimulating the muscle protein synthesis rate."

In a rare study of women at the University of Alabama (Journal of Clinical Endocrinology and Metabolism, v. 85, 2000, pp. 4476-80) they found the same results in postmenopausal women. "Total lean mass and leg lean mass were significantly correlated with free testosterone." Remember that we are talking about the normal ranges for postmenopausal women for free testosterone and the women in the higher normal ranges were slimmer and had more lean muscle mass and less fat mass. Women who have hyper levels of testosterone and DHEA outside of the normal range have a condition called "androgenicity" and need to lower those levels.

At the Universtiy of Umea in Sweden (International Journal of Obesity, v. 25, 2001, pp. 98-105) both men and women were finally studied together. In fact, both pre- and postmenopausal women were studied for even more reliable results. They found that in non-obese men and women that the higher the testosterone level the lower the leptin level. Remember that lower leptin levels are desirable and correlated with slimness. "The authors conclude that low leptin levels are associated with androgenicity in non-obese men and women and that the direction of this association is dependent on gender and body fat distribution."

FEMALE BODY FAT PERCENTAGE WITH AGE

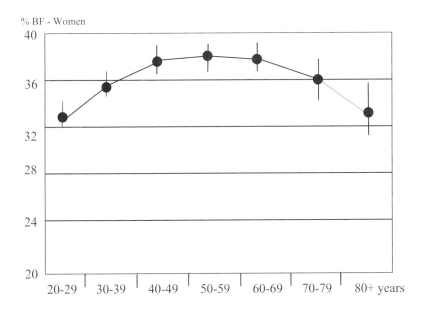

[American Journal of Clinical Nutrition v. 78 (2003)]
MALE BODY FAT PERCENTAGE WITH AGE

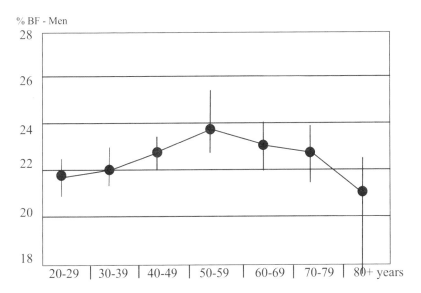

To further prove that higher testosterone levels equate with lower leptin levels and more muscle mass and less body fat we look to the University of Essen in Germany (Journal of Clinical Endocrinology & Metabolism, v. 82, 1997, pp. 407-13) "Testosterone Substitution Normalizes Elevated Serum Leptin Levels in Hypogonadal Men". Unfortunately, they used both injections of 250 mg of toxic enanthate every three weeks or a subcutaneous implantation of 1,200 mg of natural crystalline testosterone. At least the implant is natural testosterone and not some artificial salt ester. This relationship was verified at the University of Munster (Clinical Endocrinology v. 47, 1997, pp.237-40). "However, hypogonadal patients who were selected for low testosterone serum levels had significantly higher leptin serum levels and significantly higher BMI. MLR analysis revealed a significant independent association of leptin with testosterone serum levels and with BMI."

Obviously we need more research with regard to women. The same advice on diet and lifestyle applies for maintaining slimness as in every other chapter in this book. Men need to keep the youthful levels they enjoyed at about the age of thirty. Women need to keep the youthful levels while avoiding excessive ones. You must balance your other basic hormone levels (see Chapter 17 for more about this) for optimum benefits. You can see by the above charts how body fat rises in both American men and women until about the age of sixty. After the age of sixty it falls due to failing health and the inability of the body to maintain itself.

Ironically we have low body fat in our eighties, but it certainly isn't due to good diet and exercise! Women average about 34 percent body fat while men average about 23 percent. Women therefore maintain about 50 percent more adipose tissue. Americans are literally the fattest people on earth as you can see by the above charts. You'll find that people in Third World countries will have about one third less fat on their bodies due to less food available, less animal foods available and harder physical work to survive.

Chapter 16: Exercise and Strength

As one would expect, there is a large body of research regarding the effect of exercise on male testosterone levels, but very little on females. Also, the studies are often contradictory, and come with up varying results. The bottom line is that exercise helps *normalize* hormone levels and that certainly includes testosterone. This is especially true with women since they can have excessive as well as deficient levels. Having balanced hormone levels makes us stronger and gives us more endurance as well. One major reason that Americans have such out-of-sync hormone levels is our extreme inactivity. Regular exercise will help lower excessive hormone levels and raise deficient ones. Overtraining, however, such as with Olympic athletes or marathon runners is deleterious and hurts our health in the long run.

At the Baltimore branch of the National Institutes of Health (American Journal of Physiology, v. 283, 2002, pp. E284-94) the doctors were smart enough to study the free testosterone level of men. "Free Testosterone Index with Fat Free Mass and Strength in Aging Men". They found that the higher the free testosterone level was a very good predictor of muscle strength in men ranging in age from 24-90. "Muscle mass and strength losses during aging may be associated with declining levels of serum testosterone in men." They found also that the men with higher testosterone had more muscle mass and less body fat. They refer to many other studies that found the same results. They also refer to other research where supplemental testosterone in hypogonadal men resulted in more strength and more lean muscle mass. This was a most sophisticated study in great detail with fifty references.

An earlier study also published in the American Journal of Physiology (v. 282, 2002, pp. E601-7) at the University of Texas gave men with low testosterone injections of salts. Despite using the wrong type in the wrong way, they still elicited powerful results in six months. "Older men receiving testosterone increased total leg lean body mass, muscle volume, and leg and arm muscle strength." Imagine the results they would have gotten from using natural sublingual or transdermal testosterone.

The doctors at UCLA in Torrance (Journal of Clinical Endocrinology & Metabolism, v. 85, 2000, pp. 2839-53) were sophisticated enough to use transdermal gel in men. "Transdermal Testosterone Gel Improves Muscle Strength and Body Composition Parameters in Hypogonadal Men." They found the usual increases in fat free mass, decreases in body fat, and impressive increases in strength and muscle size by also having the men exercise. "Mean muscle strength in the leg press exercise increases by 11-13 kg in all treatment groups by ninety days. Moderate increases were also observed in arm/chest muscle strength." The many other benefits these men got are discussed in other chapters. This is good science by good researchers.

More modern doctors at the University of Connecticut (Journals of Gerontology, v. 56A, 2001, pp. M266-72) used transdermal testosterone patches (5 mg delivered daily) on elderly men (average age 76) for one year. Estrogen (estradiol and estrone) levels, PSA levels and prostate volume basically remained the same. Their free, unbound levels of testosterone rose 75 percent from 3.2 nM to 5.6nM. "Strength increased 38 percent in the testosterone group." Body fat decreased significantly while lean body mass (muscle) increased as did their bone mineral density. Many other biological parameters were measured and this was a very professional long-term study.

It is true that exercise will improve hormone levels dramatically for a few hours. We must remember this is a temporary phenomenon. But, it is very indicative of the power of exercise to balance our hormone levels. If you exercise regularly you will make permanent changes as long as you continue your program. At the University of Kanazawa in Japan (Horumon to Rinsho, v. 40, 1992, pp. 715-23) young men (average age of 24) exercised vigorously on stationary bicycles. Their growth hormone went up an amazing 1,850 percent! Their parathyroid hormone went up 182 percent. Their testosterone went up a full 110 percent or more than double. Vitamin D3, free T3, and free T4 all doubled. Insulin and C-reactive peptide both fell. This was an exceptionally intricate and unique study where dozens of such parameters were studied.

Studies at the University of Texas (Journal of Laboratory and Clinical Medicine, v. 34, 1999, pp. 7-10) found strength benefits from both supplemental testosterone and growth hormone (rhGH). "In summary, testosterone administration to human patients will increase muscle strength and muscle protein synthesis and may stimulate intramuscular IFG-1 system. rhGH administration to human patients will improve muscle strength in GH-deficient adults and improve body composition in older individuals and GH-deficient adults."

Fortunately at the University of Jyvaskyla in Finland (Acta Physiologica Scandinavia, v. 148, 1993, pp. 199-207) women were included in such studies! Testosterone tends to fall in women as they age especially prior to menopause. "In the females significant positive correlations were observed between the individual values in serum testosterone concentration and the values both in the muscle cross sectional area (CSA) and in maximal force (physical strength). The present results imply that the decreasing basic level of blood testosterone over the years in aging people, especially in females, may lead to decreasing anabolic effects on muscles thus having an association with age-related declines in the maximal voluntary neuromuscular performance capacity in aging people." They said further, "In the female subjects the individual values in serum testosterone correlated significantly with the individual values of maximal force, and with the individual values of maximal rate of force production as well as with the individual values of the CSA of older females." The next year (Acta Physiologica Scandinavia, v. 150, pp. 211-19) a similar study was done. Serum testosterone went up and cortisol fell in both sexes during the 12-week training. "The present findings demonstrate that considerable gains may take place in strength during progressive strength training both in middle-aged and elderly people." The findings also point out the importance of the anabolic hormonal level for the trainability of muscle strength of an individual during prolonged strength training especially in elderly males and females."

The scientists at Pennsylvania State University also realized testosterone is important for women (European Journal of Applied Physiology, v. .78, 1998, pp. 69-76). Untrained women were given a three-stage program of resistance exercise (weight lifting). Testosterone and growth hormone went up in the women while cortisol fell. "These data illustrate that untrained individuals may exhibit early-phase endocrine adaptations during a resistance training program. These hormonal adaptations may influence and help to mediate other adaptations in the nervous system and muscle fibers." Research such as this shows women as well as men normalize and improve their entire endocrine balance with regular exercise in a very short time.

Female adolescent athletes were studied at Southeastern Lousiana University (European Journal of Applied Physiology, v. 86, 2001, pp. 85-91). "It appears therefore, that DHEA, DHEA-S, ... testosterone, and leptin concentrations increase in response to running in adolescent female runners. Data also suggest that training and/or maturation increases resting testosterone concentra-tions and testosterone responses to running in adolescent female runners during a training session." Again, exercise improves the hormonal profile in women of all ages including teenagers.

We have seen how scant the research is for women and there is no reason to go on with the hundreds of studies for men. Regular exercise is important to maintaining hormonal balance. Exercise will help lower those that are too high and raise those that are too low. If you are low in any hormones it is not enough to simply take a supplement. Life extension means living a healthy life style, not just taking supplements. You must eat well, exercise regularly and avoid bad habits (such as alcohol) that will unbalance your endocrine system. Maintaining youthful levels of all your basic hormones will make you more physically fit and give you more endurance and strength throughout your life.

Your Basic 14 Hormones

- **Testosterone**
- **Androstenedione**
- **Pregnenolone**
- **DHEA**
- **Melatonin**
- **Progesterone**
- **Estradiol**
- **Estrone**
- **Estriol**
- **T3**
- **T4**
- **Growth Hormone**
- **Insulin**
- **Cortisol**

People need to balance their basic fourteen hormones as much as possible in order to prevent and cure illness, enjoy full health and have long life. If there is one basic thing to repeat over and over, it is that all *our hormones work together* in concert and they all must be at youthful levels as much as possible. Do not just be concerned with testosterone or any other hormone by itself without including all the others that work together with it.

The basic other thirteen hormones include DHEA, pregnenolone, melatonin, androstenedione, progesterone, estriol, estrone, cortisol, estradiol, T3, T4, insulin, and growth hormone. (Cholesterol is technically also a hormone and is covered in my book *Lower Cholesterol Without Drugs*.) Growth hormone testing still must be performed by a doctor using a blood draw. Soon we will have a saliva test for this as well.

DHEA is very important, basic and powerful. The benefits of having a youthful DHEA level are far too numerous to mention. There are hundreds of impressive published clinical studies in men and women of all ages. Unfortunately, many of these studies did not measure the patients to see if they were deficient. People were often given excessive 50 mg or higher doses — even women. Such irresponsible science is simply inexcusable. Women have lower levels of DHEA and need to take less as a supplement. Never, never take DHEA without first testing your blood (either free DHEA or DHEA-S) or saliva levels to see if you are deficient. Our levels usually start to fall about the age of forty and keep falling until we die. Some people, especially women, can however have high-normal or even hyper DHEA levels as they age. Thus, you cannot just assume you are deficient because you are forty or older. Men can take 25 mg daily if they are low and check their level after six months to see if this is the correct dose. Women can take 12.5 mg (half tablets) and check their level the same way. Do not accept a normal level for your age, but rather keep the youthful level you had about the age of thirty.

Pregnenolone is the basic source of all the other sex hormones, but is the "forgotten" or "orphan" hormone because we

94

know so little about it. This is *the* basic brain, memory, learning and cognition hormone, yet there has been almost no research done on it. What knowledge we do have is overwhelmingly positive and shows great promise for supplementation in people who need it. Doctors do not know nor care about pregnenolone - this includes endocrinologists and neurologists amazingly enough. Our levels generally fall at about the age of 35-40 for both men and women and then stabilize and remain low. Men over the age of forty can take 50 mg a day and check their levels after, say, six months and women over forty can take 25 mg a day and do the same check. Taking 100 mg of PS (phosphatidyl serine) and 500 mg of acetyl-L-carnitine along with your pregnenolone is an effective way of avoiding senility, memory loss, impaired cognition, and Alzheimer's.

Melatonin is truly a miraculous hormone that regulates our biological aging clock. The media will tell you this is merely good for jet lag! The truth is that melatonin is being studied for cancer prevention and treatment among many other benefits. Our levels fall from the time we leave our teenage years and keep falling until we die. A good dose is 3 mg if you are over forty and you can test your levels (at 3:00 AM with saliva) after, say, six months to see if this is the correct dose. Some people have naturally high levels and cannot take melatonin until they reach their fifties or sixties, so be sure to test your level. Some life extension advocates advise taking large doses of 5-10 mg, which is very irresponsible. As always, we are looking for youthful levels and not high, out-of-range results.

Androstenedione (and androstenediol) is the direct precursor to testosterone in both men and women. Your androstenedione level generally and basically tracks your testosterone level. It is not necessary to measure your androstenedione level unless you are a female with a suspected hyperandrogen condition. Men cannot normally have excessive androstenedione levels, just as they cannot naturally have excessive testosterone levels. Women can suffer from "androgenicity" which means they have excessive DHEA, testosterone and androstenedione levels. Such a condition causes serious problems. There seems to be no reason to try and raise low levels of androstenedione per se since they will generally go up by themselves if testosterone supplements are used.

Estriol is the "forgotten", good, or beneficial estrogen. There is very, very little published information on estriol amazingly enough. This is *the* most abundant estrogen in both men and women, comprising 80-90 percent of human estrogen, yet we know very, very little about it (and almost nothing regarding men - fortunately very few men have been found to have low estriol levels). What we do know is most impressive regarding benefits for women. Doctors, gynecologists and endocrinologists generally do not know nor care about this most abundant and basic estrogen. No U.S. pharmaceutical corporation makes an estriol product and no chain or independent pharmacies carry estriol in any form. The very few doctors who do know about it are so uneducated they generally recommend toxic, unnatural oral estriol ester salts.

The only way to use estriol is to go to a compounding pharmacist with a prescription for 100 grams of a 0.3 percent (three parts per thousand) transdermal cream or gel. This will apply 1.5 mg on the skin and 1.0 mg should be absorbed if a half gram a day is used. Sublingual estriol vegetable oil solution (1 mg per drop) would be another natural and effective means of delivery, and a compounding pharmacist could easily make this up for you. A DMSO solution could also be made (1 mg per drop), but is not legally available. There is not one single published study in the scientific literature that has measured women of different ages for their estriol level and made a chart showing normal levels! This is beyond understanding for the most basic of all human estrogens. Asian and vegetarian women have higher levels on the average. Your doctor will not know anything about estriol, but can send in a blood sample to a major lab and get your *free* (not bound) estriol (you must emphasize this) level checked. It is much easier to saliva test your level. Soon the Mexican online pharmacies are going to wake up and sell a good transdermal estriol cream or gel inexpensively and legally without a prescription. Meanwhile you have to find a sympathetic doctor who will even write a prescription for the compounding pharmacist.

96

Estrone is a powerful and potentially dangerous estrogen. Men over fifty literally have higher estrone (and estradiol) levels than their post-menopausal wives! This is frightening! Estrone deficiency in men seems almost nonexistent. Western women are generally excessive in both estrone (and estradiol) and rarely deficient. However, women with hysterectomies (one third of American women) may have a problem since their ovaries have atrophied and died even if they were not removed. You can test your free (you must emphasize this), not bound, estrone level with a blood draw or use a saliva test. If deficient and out of range women can use a naturally synthesized, bioidentical estrone tablet or cream, but never equine (horse) estrogen. You can use the patches, but they are unnecessary and very expensive. Use a compounding pharmacist for this since he will know more than the regular pharmacist

Estradiol is the most powerful and most dangerous estrogen and the least abundant percentage-wise. Estradiol deficiency in men seems almost non-existent. Women are rarely deficient in estradiol; western women are generally excessive as just mention-ed. However, after a hysterectomy there may be a deficiency of estradiol. You can measure your free (you must emphasize this), not bound, estradiol level with a blood draw or use a saliva test. If out of range women can use a naturally synthesized, bioidentical tablet or cream, just as with estrone. You can use the patches, but they are very expensive. Use a compounding pharmacist for this just as you would with estrone. Never use equine estrogens.

Men and women both need youthful levels of *pro-gesterone*. This is not a "feminizing" hormone for men. On the contrary, it opposes and balances the estrogens in both sexes. Just find a good, reliable brand of transdermal progesterone cream that contains 800-1,000 mg per two-ounce jar (400-500 mg per ounce). For women this is covered in my book *No More Horse Estrogen!* Women can use this according to their menopausal status. Men can simply use one eighth ($1/8^{th}$) teaspoon five days a week directly on their scrotum. This is covered in my book *The Natural Prostate Cure.*

Thyroid problems are epidemic in America and usually the problem is lack of hormones (hypothyroidism) rather than excessive (hyperthyroidism) ones. *T4* (L-thyroxine or Synthroid®) is usually low rather than *T3* (triiodothyronine or Cytomel®). Contrary to the usual wisdom, both Synthroid® and Cytomel® are synthesized, but bio-identical hormones, chemically identical to the ones in your body. Often naïve and uneducated naturopathic doctors will recommend Armour Thyroid, which is derived from bovine (cow) or porcine (pig) thyroid glands. The problem here is that this contains the usual 4-1 mixture of L-thyroxine and triiodothyronine. Therefore, the only people who can use this are the rare ones who are low in both. You obviously cannot use Armour Thyroid unless you are low in *both* T3 and T4. Saliva kits are available in 2004, but only (www.diagnostechs.com) one company seems to offer this service. You can also see a doctor and get a blood draw for free T3 and free T4. Do *not* let the doctor waste your time and money testing your TSH, T3 uptake or other unnecessary tests. Just get your free T3 and free T4 measured. Do not accept low normal ranges even though your doctor may tell you this is "fine" as long as you are in range. You want a healthy *youthful* range. If you are low in T4 try 50 mcg of Synthroid. If you are low in T3 try 12.5 mcg of Cytomel. If this isn't enough use more, but be careful. You can buy these legally and inexpensively from the Mexican online pharmacies without a prescription. You will probably get the most dramatic and obvious effects with thyroid hormones if you are deficient than any other hormones.

Cortisol is the stress hormone. While it is ideal to do a 24-hour cortisol test with a specimen done every six hours, you can simply do one test at 8:00 or 9:00 AM. If you are low be thankful as this is the stress hormone and low levels basically are good levels. If you are too low then only better diet, exercise, ceasing bad habits and a general change in lifestyle is going to help you. You would not want to take supplemental cortisol shots. If you are too high, again you must change your diet and lifestyle and deal with whatever stress is causing this. Balancing your other thirteen hormones will go a long way towards normalizing your cortisol levels. Again, regular exercise is vital here.

Growth hormone (somatatropin) falls as we age and almost disappears in the elderly. There are no saliva tests for GH, and you *cannot* use IGF-1 levels contrary to the popular wisdom. IGF-1 does not parallel GH, no matter what you read somewhere else. You can get a blood test at 8:00 or 9:00 A.M., but the levels of GH can vary during the day, so that these are not as reliable as are the other hormone tests. The only really accurate way to measure GH would be to take a blood draw every six hours for one day, and most people are just not able to do that. Soon we will have 24-hour GH saliva testing to give us accurate results. If you are over fifty you most probably are deficient and can use a supplement. *No OTC growth hormone supplements work.* Period. Write this down somewhere so you don't forget it. All the junk you see sold in health food stores, in catalogs, and on the Internet have no value whatsoever regardless of how well the advertising is written. The homeopathic GH is the worst fraud. Only real prescription, injectable rhGH (recombinant human) works. The problem is not only the fact it has to be injected subcutaneously (under the skin and not in your veins), but that it will cost you a minimum of $1,500 a year (Chinese Jintropin®) to buy 10 mg (which is 30 IU) of rhGH every month. Saizen® and others will cost you about $3,600 a year minimum.

These are available from the foreign online pharmacies legally by registered mail. (If you use growth hormone as a nasal spray you would need ten times as much.) All the expensive and exotic peptides like hexarelin have been extensively tested in humans, but have all failed for one reason or another. We are years away from success with such synthetic secretagogues, especially in a practical, convenient, easy to use nasal spray. They will still be expensive when they do become available. Unless you're willing to pay at least $1,500 a year and inject this at least twice a week (4 IU each time) you cannot benefit from this. You could dissolve ten mg (30 IU) of freeze dried rhGH in 60 drops of DMSO (keep it refrigerated after doing so) and use two drops a day sublingually instead of injecting it. Such sublingual use of 1 IU a day needs clinical research however and is not legally available.

Americans have an epidemic of blood sugar problems especially *insulin* resistance, diabetes and hypoglycemia. "Insulin resistance" means that the insulin we produce does not get accepted by the receptor cells so in order to compensate, we produce higher amounts. Testing your insulin or your blood sugar may not tell you much. You should take a simple and inexpensive GTT (glucose tolerance test) where you drink a measured dose of glucose solution, and a blood draw is taken two hours later to see if your blood sugar has normalized. If you are insulin resistant or have any blood sugar dysmetabolism you have to change your diet and lifestyle. As long as your pancreas is intact this can be very easy to do with very good results. You must cut down on meat and fats, take dairy out of your life, not eat refined grains, and eat no fruit, sugars or sweeteners whatsoever including honey, molasses, etc. There are a variety of supplements that will help you including lipoic acid, CoQ10, beta glucan, and a complete mineral supplement. In 2005 my book *The Natural Diabetes Cure* will be published.

Again, all your basic hormones should be balanced as they all work together in concert. Just raising your testosterone when some of your other hormones are deficient is just not going to give you the effects you want or can get. It may seem arduous to try and test all your basic hormones and balance them, but the more you do the more benefits you will get. Thirteen of the fourteen can be saliva tested very inexpensively and one doctor's visit can take care of rhGH. Except for growth hormone, none of them are expensive. All are available legally under U.S. Code Section 21, Section 331 for personal use (up to fifty dosage units) imported by mail or coming back into the country.

Other Books By Safe Goods

The Natural Prostate Cure- Roger Mason	$ 6.95 US $10.95 CAN
No More Horse Estrogen!- Roger Mason	$ 7.95 US $11.95 CAN
Zen Macrobiotics for Americans- Roger Mason	$ 7.95 US $11.95 CAN
Lower Cholesterol Without Drugs- Roger Mason	$ 6.95 US $10.95 CAN
What is Beta Glucan? - Roger Mason	$ 4.95 US $ 7.95 CAN
The Minerals You Need- Roger Mason	$ 4.95 US $ 7.95 CAN
The Natural Diabetes Cure- Roger Mason (due in 2005)	
Dr. Vagnini's Healthy Heart Plan- Dr Vagnini	$16.95 US $24.95 CAN
Overcoming Senior Moments-Anderson/Meiser	$ 7.95 US $11.95 CAN
Natural Born Fatburners-Dr. Redmon	$14.95 US $22.95 CAN
Eye Care Naturally-Dr. Geiger	$ 8.95 US $12.95 CAN
Cancer Disarmed Expanded-Nina Anderson	$ 7.95 US $11.95 CAN
Low Carb and Beyond –Anderson/Peiper	$ 9.95 US $12.95 CAN
ADD, The Natural Approach-Anderson/Peiper	$ 4.95 US $ 7.95 CAN
2012 Airborne Prophecy-Nina Anderson	$16.95 US $24.95 CAN

U.S. toll free (888) NATURE-1 (628-8731)
www.safegoodspub.com
Safe Goods Publishing, 561 Shunpike Road, Sheffield, MA 01257